Return to the Soul of Your Child

"Soul of A Child"

By

Mary Olea Lesher M.A.E.

Mary Olea Lesher

http://gracefulroadmusic.com

Preface

This book started long ago. I recently had a transformational experience that reminded me how much our early life experiences help set who we become. I decided to put this in the book because, in effect, I inadvertently did return to the soul of my child. When I was a little one, about three years old, my birth father and mother were experiencing marital discord. I was a witness to this discord and I remember being barefooted and in a diaper trying to be very quiet. I was creeping down a dark hall and I hid under my crib. I was still sleeping in a crib. I hid under my crib in a tight little ball. I didn't have words for what I saw and heard but I was frightened. I knew my mother was in danger and instinct told me so was I. Shortly after that, my mother and father divorced. This was in the early 1950s and this was not a common thing at that time.

My mother remarried and I was raised by a stepfather who is really the only Dad I remember. As I was growing up, I would try to talk to my mother about the time I saw the scary things. That door was shut and I was never allowed to speak of it.

Years flowed along to where I am now. I thought I was free from the past. I have released and let go of so many old formats and patterns, I am actually having fun with my life! This Father's Day Sunday, I was in church and a visiting minister was sharing his childhood story. His name is Pastor Chris Peterson and was giving his message at St. Ansgar's Lutheran Church in Salinas Ca. He was an infant in his mother's arms and they were in a car accident. She lost her life protecting her baby's life. He survived the accident. He was raised by a father who had anger issues. It took him many years to forgive his father. As he shared his very personal and vulnerable story of forgiveness towards his father, a tear rolled down my cheek. Just one tear. My upbringing taught me to not cry in public.

As he continued to speak, I was having a different experience. It felt like a horizontal bar of dark, heavy energy was coming up my body from the feet up. It moved from my feet to ankles, to stomach, heart, neck, head. It felt so dark and heavy and old. I knew without words what it was. It was the unspoken fear, anger, sadness, and terror of that little three-year-old girl hiding under her crib in a tight ball. Somehow, I knew not to analyze the experience and I knew I needed to see my arms lifting up the dark energy bar over my head. In my mind, I held up the horizontal bar of dark, sad, old energy up to the cross and I released it to God. My single tear fell to the floor.

I felt one thousand pounds lighter. Whew! *What just happened?* I was wondering as I left my church to return home. I left church feeling like a new person.

I kept thinking about this experience and I knew that my work on the issue of forgiveness from the past was not finished. Previous to this experience, I thought I had made my peace with life. I am sixty-four years old—what else is there to talk about? I decided to go to a Forgiveness Workshop given by Reverend Sherry McCreary who gives wonderful workshops. revsherry@revsherry.com

She guided us through exercises and, in one of the guided exercises, I visualized the adult me taking the hand of the three-year-old me and facing "our" birth father. I spoke for both of us with my adult voice and forgave him for what I had seen so long ago. The three-year-old me did not want to see him or talk to him, but the adult Mary now spoke with full adult voice.

We forgave my birth father for his actions. His face faded away and in the guided mediation, I picked up the little Mary and held her in my arms. I folded her into my heart. I think I maybe done now with this old energy from the past. It was a part of who I became but now I am free of the old, sad, dark feelings that my three-year-old self had no words for. Writing this book helped me trigger this experience for me. As you read *Return to the Soul of Your Child*, you may find tools that you can use in your own life's journey.

Mary Olea Lesher
Author

The Purpose of This Book

The purpose of this book is to share eye-opening, potentially inspiring insights. Key and crucial insights that may guide the reader to the greatest of all gifts, which, in this case, is finding your life's purpose. Sometimes, we have life experiences that set our lives on other purposes other than our true purpose in life.

The reason behind the need for this book is clear: simply put, sometimes, we just have life experiences that set our lives on other purposes other than our true purpose in life. This, of course, can lead to frustration, despair, depression, and addiction to all types of self-numbing actions and or substances. Thus, finding that ultimate life-enlivening soul purpose is part of the great mysteries of life.

There are many routes to one's purpose. There are many ways to find your purpose. *Return to the Soul of Your Child* is just one of them. In my case, I found a gift that was in me and I bumped into that purpose, almost as if it had been looking for me and had finally caught me. To embrace that life-giving purpose, I had to learn to look at myself differently from the way I had been "personally formatted" by my life experiences. I am a new person from the person formally noted as unmusical. I am a musician, and it brings great joy to my life to share my music. I have had a lot of joy with my "gift," and I know in my heart there are many other people—women, men, girls, and boys—who have gifts that they might find if I share my story.

To lay some groundwork for you as a reader, I will tell you a little about my own background as a traveler on life's road. I was a baby boomer. Boom. This war ripped apart many lives. The war over, men and women who had their lives diverted by the Second World War returned home to the States to restart their personal lives. Some separations were as long as four years, as with the case of my parents. When these people reunited, Baby Boomers were born!

Women returned to the United States after serving actively in the war effort, while men returned looking for jobs to support their growing family. Women who had been active in work and service during the war were reassigned to domestic, caretaker roles of the late

1940s and into the 1950s. Women's lib had not yet become an active part of our society. Women were encouraged to return to the domestic role previously assigned to them by society.

Overall, women did not work outside the home. The "ideal" picture of American life was a working father as head of the house, and a stay-at-home mother. It took several decades and women's liberation to change this for more women. Now, it is totally acceptable for a mother to work outside the home. I was one of these little baby boomers. The format I was given was the one that women were given at that time.

I was born in 1948. As a female, I was, for all intents and purposes, an unremarkable child. What did it mean to be born in 1948? Well, roles were definitely stereotypical for girls and boys. If you were a boy, you were dressed in baby boy blue and given little cars and little guns, and the language that surrounded you was different from the one if you were born a little girl.

My life experience was that of a little girl. Little girls in 1948 were dressed in baby pink. They were given baby dolls to play with, little ironing boards, and encouraged to become wives and, eventually, mommies! The language of that era was different for females and males from it is now. That is just the way it was.

Women only had the vote in the United States in 1923! Women still were learning to find their voice. Women's lib had not yet begun. If you were a girl, the messages you received in school and at home were messages that prepared you for a domestic role.

That was a given if you were a little girl. That was your vision of who you would be and what you should do with your life. No one argued with it at that time, and there was not a lot of dialogue about more opportunity for women. Women were brought up to be caretakers, wives, and mothers. There is your pink dress, there is your baby doll! That is what you really want to do with your life! That was the assigned societal role at the time. That is just the way it was.

The window of time that I entered life through had messages for me to the effect that I was first of all a girl. Secondly, I was a middle-of-the-road person. I was a C student academically, but a very sweet person. I would be a good wife and mother. I was expected to be good, well-behaved, and compliant. I can remember as a little girl seeing little boys running around outside with their shirts off in the summer! I wanted to take my shirt off, too, and run around freely and play in the sun. My mother said, "Mary, you are a little girl. Little girls have to wear their shirts." I really wanted to be a little boy! Why did I have to be a little girl and wear my shirt? Oh, well, I wore my shirt but I still did go out to play! The world was different then and opportunities to develop talents for women and men were different then. It wasn't anything personal, it was just the time, place, and culture that existed at the time, and I was being formatted by it as surely as we are all formatted by our culture now.

My mother divorced my birth father when I was three years old. In 1951, this was rare. I remember chaotic marital discord and shortly after that, she and I, holding her hand, left that life setting. We lived with various relatives and, in a while, she met my stepfather. He was a military man. She married him. He is the dad I remember. I haven't seen or heard from my birth father since I was very little.

My stepfather was very strict, but our life was well ordered. He ruled his household with an iron hand. He was very disciplined, but he never struck us. I remember growing up and when we were "talked" to, it seemed we were barked at. It was the way children used to be talked to. When you parents said "Jump!" you jumped! Children used to be seen and not heard. Why was it that way? I think it was because of the time that every one had come through. If you were raised in the Depression and struggled for existence, you didn't waste time on saying things more than once. Also, coming through the wars changed the way people looked at life. There was a strict urgency in the way children were raised. Children did as they were told—there was not an option to be disrespectful. Children were also told they were being provided with a roof over their heads and food to eat every day. They were reminded to be thankful for that provision and respectful toward their parents. There was not a sense of entitlement or that anyone owed you anything. Respect towards your parents was an inherent part of the culture in the window of time that I entered the world. Parents of that era were not worried about being their children's best friend and having their children's friends think they were cool. Parents held a strict and guiding hand over their children's lives. It was a different time and place. "Yes, Sir" and "Yes, Ma'am," "No, Sir" and "No, Ma'am" were the order of the day. It didn't seem so strange then.

What is good about me as a person I learned from my "step" father. I do not think of him as my stepfather but my real father. He was very disciplined and had a will of iron. He would not give up on something once he started it. He passed away when he was ninety years old. He and my mother were married for fifty-two years. In fact, when my mother passed away, only a month and a day later, he went to heaven to join her. They had been gone for eight years now.

Divorce in 1951 was frowned upon. Now, it is different in our culture and it is accepted in a more compassionate way. In 1951, there had to be something wrong with a couple if they divorced. No matter what the circumstances or the reasons a person left a relationship, it was not okay! I remember growing up with my sister and going to school and being asked, "Why do you have a different last name from your sister's?" It was frequently an awkward feeling to have to try and explain why my name was different. I was just a kid and it felt awkward. I always had the feeling that if people's parents were not divorced, they seemed smug about themselves and their lives. You know what it feels like to have someone "look down their nose at you"? "Well, my parents are not divorced!" What do you say when you are a little kid and you really can't explain why your parents got divorced? You were only three years old when it happened. The world is much more compassionate about divorced people now.

What did I mean by being an unremarkable child? When I was growing up a girl in the 1950s, I remember being given ballet lessons and piano lessons. I never impressed my teachers. My early attempts to play piano were discouraged. Instead of giving messages to just keep on trying, I was told, "You have no musical ability." A piano teacher I took lessons from told my parents they were wasting their money on my lessons. That took care of that. "Take typing and shorthand. You will be a good wife and mother." The goal of the time I was being raised in was to prepare you for a domestic role. That was the big life goal and that was what most women wanted to prepare themselves for. If you were lucky enough to be pretty, you didn't have to worry about being good in math. The girls who needed to be smart were the ones who didn't have good looks. I also heard things like, "Boys don't make passes at girls who wear glasses." I have worn glasses since the fourth grade! Oh, well, my life has gone on nonetheless! I remember in high school that the classes girls were encouraged to attend were homemaking and sewing. There were exciting groups like Latin Club and Kayettes. This was a lifetime ago! I remember the girls club, the Kayettes, had a theme song that went something like this: "A man without a Kayette is like a ship upon the sand, he's like a boat without a rudder, he's like a ship without a sail. A man without a Kayette is like a boat upon the sand, but there is one thing worse in the universe, oh, it's a Kayette, oh, it's a Kayette, oh, it's a Kayette without a man! That's the truth!" We sang it at our meetings and we thought that was so cool! Ha! Are you gagging yet? That was the goal young women were given!

I was the recipient of many life messages that diminished rather than supported growth. My musical website http://gracefulroadmusic.com bears witness to another story.

These early messages set the pattern in my life that forged my sense of self. With the early message of my childhood, I married at eighteen and a half years old. I began my adult journey.

When my husband and I had been married for four months, he was drafted into military service to serve in the war in Vietnam. This happened to thousands of people in those times. If you were not in college or you didn't have rich parents, you probably had a good chance of being drafted. The year was 1966 and the war was escalating. He left our home to be trained and sent to Vietnam. He was gone for two years.

We had very brief contact when he was in military service. When we did see each other, it was for very short leaves and then he would have to return to military service. The saddest part of seeing him was to see him leave again. I would know that there was a good chance I would not see him alive again. He saw friends come home in body bags or maimed in battle. He was one of the lucky ones. He came home alive and unharmed. It was a politically unpopular war. One of the "fun" ways to harass the wives of the men serving in this politically incorrect war was to call them on the phone at night and tell them their husbands had been killed in service. I didn't answer the phone at night. I prayed there would not be a knock on the door with two uniformed Army personnel to tell me the sad news of my husband's loss of life. There were thousands of people like us. We were not the exception to the rule.

My husband returned home safe and sound in 1968. We started our married life together again. While he was gone, I tried to save up for a new car and a house. We had a little nest egg when he came home. A few years passed and we started our family.

My husband of forty-six years and I have raised our two sons. They are grown now. Adults with their own lives. I barked at them when they grew up. I did modify the life messages I gave them. They both lead productive adult lives. They were patterned by my words to become who they are.

In 1972, when our first child was born, women who were obviously expecting did not work in the workplace. I quit my bank job when I was six months pregnant. In the wait for our baby, I had an urge to play the guitar. Some women want pickles and ice cream. Some women want watermelon. I wanted to play the guitar. "I want a guitar," I told my husband. "Why?" "I don't know! I just want to play guitar." He bought me my first guitar. It was a small $15.00 child-sized guitar. That's when it all started. Music said "Hello" to me. I took a summer course shortly before our son was born. I happily waddled out of class with three or four guitar chords. I was totally happy! Little songs started to happen, but that is a different story. Check out my musical website! http://gracefulroadmusic.com

My songs resided in spaghetti-stained manila folder in my kitchen. I knew a small group of guitar chords and when my baby was asleep, I would strum my guitar. Words and music "happened". I would write down the words and put the chord names above the words. I would sing the melodies into a tape recorder to remember them. I did not read a note of music. Remember? I was told I was not musical. Hmmm?

The best part of my guitar fun was that it was my hobby and it was my fun. I didn't care!

I had a girl friend who knew how to write out music. I traded her babysitting for scoring. I figured out how to copyright my songs. I started to really want to know how to read music.

I had a great desire to read music. Music led me to junior college. I eventually acquired an associate of arts degree. I ended up teaching a lot of guitar and found out I was better that mediocre. I was a bright person and I loved learning! Long story short, I eventually acquired a bachelor's degree at the age of forty-nine and teaching credential at the age of fifty. I began teaching my first elementary school class at the age of fifty.

My life had taught me to be kinder with my words than I had experienced. My teaching career allowed me to experience human consciousness in broader sense. I became aware of the power of words and used them to guide student effort.

My journey to acquire a teaching degree at a relatively late age took years of effort in-between wash loads. I remember when I started to go to a local junior college, my sons in grade school would look at me packing up my book bag and say, "Mom, you don't even have to go to school, but you do." The school bus would stop to pick them up and when they left for school, I left for school. I was lucky to be able to take one or two classes a semester. It was very slow going. It was a class at a time over time.

I also remember standing in line holding a young child to register for a music class. I really wanted to learn to read music. I remember the person helping students to register wanted to dismiss me as a person who was wasting his time. "You can't just take music classes," this person told me. I started out with music classes and eventually learned to get a counselor to help me set my course through junior college. I remember thinking that I would be so happy to read music and the idea of an AA degree seemed impossible to me at the time. I am a very persistent person and I just kept on keeping on.

This is not the best way to go to college, but it is the way that I did it. Once you have family responsibilities, your educational journey is different. I actually didn't push myself harder to get my teaching degree until my children were in their late teens.

They were older and more independent, and it was easier for me to be gone longer periods of time at school. When I finished junior college, I had to wait a number of years before I transferred to a college that would prepare me to become a school teacher. I was in my middle forties when I tackled this part of my educational journey. I transferred to the closest school that I could attend. It was San Jose State University. I remember commuting two thousand miles a month to my classes. I would get up at 4:00 a.m. in the morning and leave by 5:00 a.m. I would park in the parking garage and get to class. Then I would make a beeline for home to teach guitar at a local music store and eventually a junior college. Then I would go home to study for my next day's classes and then go to bed and do it all over again.

There was a short period of time that my oldest son and I actually commuted to the same college together. Whoever had a test to study for didn't have to drive. I know it had to be a drag to see your mother at the same school as you packing her backpack around. He studied in a different part of the campus so we pretty much didn't see much of each other. There were times I was so tired I just wanted to cry but I didn't, I had too much work to do.

I remember giving my son the advice that no one was there to give to me. I told him get a good counselor and only take classes that you need. Don't waste time taking classes that don't add up to your degree. That is one reason it took me so long to get my B.A. degree in education. I had to learn how to play the academic game. My son told me, "Mom, I'm not waiting for you to graduate!" He finished his first B.A. in four years and was on his way to his adult life.

I was very happy when California State University of Monterey Bay opened up in my area in 1995. I applied to the school and waited for over a year to be accepted as a student there. Transferring from the school I was going to would extend my educational journey, but I wouldn't have the long commute and could take a full load of academic classes. When I started to attend CSUMB, there were a little over five hundred students. It was a huge change from a campus with over twenty-five thousand students. Now, of course, there are several thousand students attending there.

I was on fire to finish school and become a classroom teacher. I kept teaching guitar to help pay for school and carried a full load of classes. I also took care of my home and family. When I graduated at the age of forty-nine years old with my bachelor's degree, it was one of the happiest days in my adult life. Education was my major and music was my minor. I had a year to go to get my teacher's credential and then I could enter the classroom as a classroom teacher. I was fifty when I achieved that.

The twelve and a half years that I taught in the public school classroom taught me many things about people in general. Every one is from a different background and has different ways to look at life. I did learn that overall, children respond to positive messages and will generally try and make more of an effort when encouraged by positive words. My service as a classroom teacher piqued my interest in self-efficacy.

In my early fifties, I started to work on my master's degree. It took me longer than I wanted to complete it because I dropped out of the study program at the end of my parents' lives. I knew they needed me on the weekends and I found that it was too difficult to work full time as a teacher and take master classes and also to be there in an effective way for my parents. I did not want to have any regrets when they passed away. I know I was there for them as much as I could be and I am glad I did what I could for them. They both died in 2004. My mother was eighty years old and a month and a day after she passed away, my father died at the age of ninety. It was an emotionally sad time for me. I continued to teach. I told my husband that I had lost my drive to finish my master's degree. He told me, "Finish what you started." The wind had been taken out of my sail by my parent's deaths. I reluctantly went back to school and worked on my master's degree one class at a time. My sons were grown by now and out of the house. I would get up and go to teach, leave school, and go to my class. I would drive home at ten p.m. When I got home, I would work on homework until twelve p.m. or one a.m. Then, I would go to bed, get up at 5:00 or 6:00 a.m., and start all over again. I completed my master's study in 2008. My health started to indicate to me that I had driven myself a little too hard. The winter of 2008, I got pneumonia and missed several weeks at the end of that school year. My health started to tell me that public school teaching was demanding too much from me. I retired from teaching public school in 2010. Working with one hundred elementary school children a day wore me down.

My interest in student self-efficacy and the drive to change and grow led me to acquire a master's degree in education at the age of sixty. Two short years later, my health informed me that my twelve-and-a-half-year teaching career was over. That has led me to this book.

How can we effectively become more of who we really are?

How can we effectively become more of who we really are? What can help us return to the soul of our own child within and how do we work with ourselves and other children in our lives to experience more of our unlimited self?

Return to the Soul of Your Child **suggests ways of communication that may transform your life experiences.**

Introduction

This book embodies the *soul of a child*, which was the author's original intention when teaching in the public school settings she retired from. Her master's work references Albert Bandura and Leve Vygotsky. The work is available for educators, parents, and all others to access at the C.S.U/M/B. Library archives. http://library2.csumb.edu/capstone/world/2008/lesher_mary.pdf This link will take you directly to the study and you may access it, use it, print it out, and share it!

My Mediated Language Scaffold is based on scholarly studies, but to take the idea of language scaffold out of the classroom and into contemporary life will expand its service beyond children to all of us. We all need to consider the language that we utilize in our daily life transactions. Once I retired from teaching in the public school classroom, I felt like I had not finished the conversation I had started with my master's study. It has taken me a lifetime to analyze my own journey and see that, really, if we reformat the way we think about ourselves, we can change our life experience. It took me a long time to accept that I have musical abilities and to use them joyfully! Why weren't words there in my younger life to encourage me? I don't know. What I do know is that the way we are spoken to and the way we speak to ourselves and others have an effect on our lives. This is exciting to me because I now know that I can take the template of my mind and change it. I am the scriptwriter and it is my journey. It is also fun to share this with others because I know there are many other people like me who can also open their own minds to their own potential and explore it. Enjoy the adventure of your own life!

It will benefit the creator of the scaffold with language that will support personal growth for themselves and for those that are affected by them and their language. It will transform personal relationships and business relationships. Every one of us has access to a quiet inner place where we talk to ourselves. I like to think of it as my personal inner garden. I can go to my garden to find inspiration, quiet and restoration from life's busy demands. As you work with these ideas, go into your personal garden and ask yourself any questions that will lead you to greater personal expression and growth in your personal life. You may pause to ponder that you have never stopped to build yourself an inner garden. Do so now. What does it look like? Where are you sitting? Create it as you think about it. It is there to welcome you and it is for you to be able to find your own inner peace. It is here you will begin to consider the ideas about *Return to the Soul of Your Child.*

Think about these ideas:

We are all matrixes of conditioned responses.
Get over yourself.
Get over everyone else.
Have no attachments to outcome!
Stand free mentally in space and time.

To become aware of one's personal matrix of conditioned responses may give you more compassion towards the human experience and condition. It may allow the observer to be free from judgments.

What has made you who you are?

Every life experience, every personal habit you have acquired over time. As years fly by, acquired patterns, habits seem to have a life of their own. They become deeply embedded. Look at your personal matrix and observe it without judgment. You are who you are because...? Numerous reasons surround the mystery of who you are. They are yours to discover!

Look at your acquired matrix with great compassion and stand free of it without judgment. One of the gifts we can give ourselves if we choose is to become aware of our patterned matrix and reformat it. Another gift we can give ourselves and everyone else is to become aware of the power of our words, thoughts in resetting our own personal matrix. If you really become aware, help set the matrix pattern of little souls that follow you into your lives. Give them the gift of transformational, empowering life messages. Guide them with temperance but supportive structures as they form their personal matrix. The words that surround them, the daily life messages they hear embed themselves as their personal truths.

These personal life truths will give them scaffolds upon which they springboard into life.

Soul of a Child

The Soul of a child
Is meek and mild
How can we help it grow?
Use words of kindness
Cruel words bind us and
Keep us from the flow.

How do we touch the *soul* of a *child*? The language that surrounds us from the time we are born formats our mental picture of who we think we are. The inherently unlimited self that we all are is deep with each soul. How do we reach this part of self and invite it to manifest its unlimited gifts?

Think about the language that has surrounded you since you were born. Was that language kind and loving? Did it invite you into a wonderful, creative mental space that allowed you to discover the great adventure of your own consciousness? Review this language that has surrounded you like an ocean of words. Whatever the language, you can learn a new way to speak to yourself, to others, and most importantly, to all children who are a part of your life experience. How do we invite children to activate their unlimited self? We learn to surround them with language that is mediated with the awareness that the children format themselves with this language.

How do you greet your children? Good morning, beautiful child! Let's have a great day! What is the personal pattern that you are creating with your words to surround your unlimited child to manifest their gifts and themselves? Think about it and if you do not like what you see, explicitly create a new language for your child and your life that will broaden their creative experience as a person and yours as well.

Claim Your Power Now!

- An Active Learner sits up straight.
- An Active Learner calms down inside.
- An Active Learner opens up their mind.
- An Active Learner claims their power to learn.
- An Active Learner tries to do the learning task.
- An Active Learner knows that it is their responsibility to learn!
- Go Active Learners!
- You are the future!

Meaningful Personal Connection

Learn to cultivate a meaningful personal connection with the young people in your life. Words alone are not enough to motivate people to become self-aware and decision makers. They must also feel a meaningful personal connection with the person guiding them with the sea of language surrounding them all of their life.

The connection you build with your young people depends upon the relationship that you have. If you are a parent, the connection will be more intimate. If you are a teacher, pastor, or a youth worker, it will have to be created carefully and within the parameters of your working relationship with that young person.

Words of praise and worthiness will build self-esteem. They also help people have more self-efficacy in their attempts to live their lives.

When we are working with children, especially, and also with one another, if we keep this in mind, we can help them as they pattern themselves with memories of who they become. We become ourselves over time. It is a process over time a step at a time. Be aware of the choices you make with your words and in your personal habits. These do set your pattern. You can reset your pattern by becoming conscious and aware and finding exactly what it is you want your patterns to be.

Return to the Soul of Your Child, the scripting of our lives—there needs to be a reformatting in this world. There is such a matrix of not supportive words, not supportive ideas that surround people. People need to rise above it and find what they do want to have as their pattern and they do want to manifest in themselves and their lives and on the canvas of their lives. Try to create a script that allows you mental awareness and self mastery and helps others to do the same. Our behaviors simply reflect the way we were conditioned in our life and the formatting that we have. It is essential to become aware of the personal formats that you allow to flow through your mind on a daily basis. Surround yourself with things that will help you manifest things you want to manifest in terms of choices in life.

When we are reflective rather than reactive, we can determine what behaviors are in place and we can also decide that we can create new ones for ourselves. We can surround ourselves with language and emotional support whether it comes from us or others who can help us to forge a new identity.

No matter whom you are sharing your life with, they are a result of patterning from their childhood, early adulthood, and into full adulthood. Consequently, they act the way they do because of those patterns. Some of them are deeply ingrained. Some of them can't even look at them. They are so much a part of who they think they are, but we can be free from those patterns if you become an observer and do some different kind of formatting in our own minds with affirmative statements. Each life is a matrix of life experiences that are fundamentally patterned by the words that surround the experiences. These make us who we are and give us our life patterns.

We conscript our life's patterns and identity from the words that surround us from childhood into adult hood. We also have the power to repattern ourselves by gaining awareness of our patterns of behavior. Self-mastery takes reflection, time, and practice to put into action new patterns of awareness of who we desire to manifest in our life. Our life is the canvas of our living. We can choose to become a different representation from what we were originally programmed to become. There are many different roads to self-mastery.

One of the shortfalls of being a human being is that what we think we perceive in others is not necessarily the total picture of that person's potentiality. That is where gaining an awareness of the power of our words can help to transform the lives of those who we have influenced. The lives of young children are greatly impacted by the words of the adults who guide their growth.

It is important for everyone in service to others to become aware of the words that they use when working with those people. Whether it is in a personal relationship, such as spouse, significant other, teacher, minister, or any service to others that communicates personal value that words be chosen to guide to more positive choices, behavior and show regard for potential in the people who are being served.

Choose words carefully when working with anyone who is impressionable. Once someone is an adult, the work changes in relationship to awareness. Once patterns of belief are scripted and set, then the people these are affecting has to become consciously aware of themselves and do the rescripting themselves. This is personal work and there are many pathways to accomplishing this. It takes time, persistence, and learning to not be judgmental in relationship to perceived flaws. A flaw is simply a repetitive pattern of behavior that is in place for a variety of reasons.

Return to the Soul of Your Child

Some of us are born into life experiences where we were supported by loving, guiding language. Others had experiences that did not provide as secure a foothold into personal growth. No matter! We continue to grow into who we are and we are all part of the divine or God. Whatever your personal references, our potential is exponential and we continue to grow whatever our ages and whatever our experiences. Our experiences led us to become who we are and that is subject to change on a moment to moment basis. When we become aware of the mechanisms of change, we can employ them to build a better life scaffold for our own life experiences.

We are the authors of our own lives and we do write the script. We are scriptwriters after all. We hear our souls call us to a new day! Our lives continue to unfold, the greatest stories ever told. We find our way there. You can grow past old patterns and into new ones. You can acquire new direction and go towards new vistas of self. The old horizon has left and a new one stretches out in front of you. You can meet and greet your gifts and cultivate them. Everything is one step at a time.

Stepping out of judgment leaves you free to grow. Everyone has been patterned by the window of time they were born into and the culture that supported their growth. They are a result of their life experiences. None of us is free from patterning. Have compassion for those who gave you your patterns because they also were patterned by their lives. Soul to soul we reach out and help each other grow. Change is a part of nature and we are a part of nature. Change is good! When we search for truth and find it, we forget to let it grow. We call it truth forever, even if it isn't so.

Diminishment Speak

There is a template of negative language that I have observed in my own life and prevalent in our culture today that I have coined a term for. I call it Diminishment Speak. It seems the language that predominates reality shows, comedy shows. The basic American Cultural Anvil enjoys this language. Its template is one of diminishment of people, places, and things. It is all around us. I hear in daily transactions every day. To overcome the influence that this has on your mindset, you have to become aware of it. This does not have to remain the language template of the new millennia. We can become aware of it and change our own use of language, to have a different influence on our life and the lives of the people we share our lives with. It is such an undercurrent of influence that it predominates the mindset of many lives. We can become aware of it and we can reroute our mental energies to do something else.

Some examples of what I am talking about would be comments that lessen a person's value on some level. There are some people whose template of language seems to come out with always a negative connotation. It may be by design or inadvertently. I also think of it as "put down city" type of talk. It seems to be an entertainment to make circumstances or people less than. Some of this is typical humor and some of it is not necessary to life's daily transactions. I am also thinking about back handed compliments. These all play a part in diminishment speak. This term is one that I have coined as I assesssed the templates of language that I am aware will help to set our personal formats. You can examine the language that you have encountered on your personal journey and make your own evaluation of it.

I personally like to use language that encourages positive support of people and situations. I am not suggesting that constructive criticism does not have its place in our growth. I am only pointing out a pattern that I see in place that I call diminishment speak.

Master Control Room

As you learn to become aware of your patterns and conditioned habits of living and thinking, you may feel overwhelmed by uncertainty. "How do I begin to repattern myself?" Self-awareness is the first step. You might want to categorize different areas of your life. You might find it helpful to picture a personal control room of life habits. On the control panel are many different switches, with on and off indicators. When you see you are looping into a patterned behavior that you no longer wish in life, enter your Master Control Room and go to the switch. Reach out and turn it off! Do this as many different times as you need to. It takes gentle persistence to change the pattern. Your self-reflection will allow you to become aware of your patterns and decide what life patterns you want to live out! You cannot change anyone's mind but your own. Your growth is within you and you are free to make changes or not.

Become aware of your patterns and change the ones that no longer serve you. Choose your words carefully and know that they are a force for good in the world. Meet and greet your unlimited self and have fun! Your consciousness is an adventure and as you explore and expand it, you will manifest more of your potential. Grow like the trees in spring.

Self-Efficacy

What is self-efficacy? The master's study that references this important concept is freely available at the California State University Bay of Monterey library archives, http://library2.csumb.edu/capstone/world/2008_mary.pdf. In layperson's terms, it is how a person has a willingness to try new tasks or behaviors based upon their own evaluation of what they think they can do. It may seem obtuse, but in reality, it is the inner gear that moves us forward to new effort in whatever area we are directing our personal efforts. It is an exciting concept in education but also transformational in personal lives.

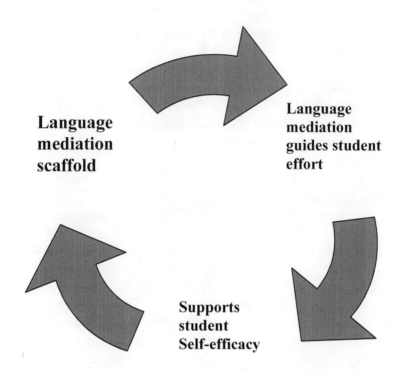

Language mediation scaffold

Language mediation guides student effort

Supports student Self-efficacy

What I observed during the course of this action research project is that the language guided students to more on-task performance. Their personal behaviors were more scholarly and their mindset appeared to be more focused in academic tasks. The following chart shows the loop from language mediation to student effort and the finally support of student self-efficacy.

There is a loop from the scaffold to the student attempt to the connection with self-efficacy. Self-efficacy is supported positively depending upon the psychological matrix of the individual student. The language of the Active Learner Mediated Language Scaffold is constructed in a way that positive influences support student self-efficacy.

The language scaffold of your life drives your efforts in many seen and unseen areas. It is empowering to gain access to this important tool of self-mastery and make it work for you in a way that you become the designer of your own life script. Be aware of the choices that you make with your words and your personal habits. These do format your mindset. You can reset your format by becoming conscious and aware and finding exactly what it is you want to have as your format. *Return to the Soul of Your Child*, the scripting of our lives, makes you the author of your own screenplay, your life. It makes you the artist of your own life's canvas. You stand with the blank canvas of every day and you paint with your words and emotions. Pick up your pen and paper, pick up brush and paint. Begin to transform your life now!

The world needs to be aware of mental reformatting. There is such a maelstrom of unsupportive words and ideas that surround people. People need to rise above it and find what they do want to have as their life pattern. They need to determine what they want to manifest in themselves. Words of praise and worthiness will build self-esteem and also help us to have more self-efficacy in our attempts to live our lives. Therefore, when we are working with children, especially, and also one another, if we keep this in mind, we can help one another to set a mental format that serves us in our lives. These mental formats help build memories of who we become. We become ourselves over time. It is a process over time, a step at a time.

Try to create a script that allows you mental awareness and self-mastery and helps others to do the same. Our behaviors simply reflect the way we were conditioned in life and the patterning that we have. It is essential to become aware of the patterning that you allow to flow through your mind on a daily basis. Surround yourself with things that will help manifest the experiences that you want to have as part of your life experience.

What you constantly think about and constantly live are the result of your language scaffold. You can redesign it and change your pattern to reflect your authentic self. You can change your pattern. It is important to be aware of how you speak and how you think because you become more self-aware. You are more present in your thoughts and in your choices. You can have a different kind of experience in life.

The great mystery speaks to us in a breeze, a dream, an imperceptible whisper, and sometimes we think we heard something.

Now, my great mystery took a two by four and kept whacking me upside the head. Hey! You are a musician! Okay. Okay, I get it. I know that now. Now, I want to share the news with everyone else that inside of them resides a beautiful undiscovered self who wants to emerge. Everyone's experience will be different. Everyone has one! Maybe you want to be a chef. Maybe you want to own a cup cake shop called Happy Eats. Maybe you want to paint pictures!

Hey, you! Listen to your potential calling you in a dream or a streaming thought. The talent, the call is in you! Do not be afraid to become more! More is part of the exponential nature of life. There is always more. The universe is expanding and so are we. Stretch and stretch some more! Go for it! Be happy! Smile! Laugh!

Let your life's adventure allow you to ponder the meaning of your formatting. Was your personal format filled with diminishment or was it full of loving supportive messages?

How do you feel in response to your life and the people around you? If you want to change that—do so. If your life is fine the way it is, enjoy it! Growing is not always comfortable. When we have to make changes in our lives, it feels strange but the outcome can be good. Life is experiential and it can become a joyful adventure. Ask yourself the question, "Who am I now?" The now of you will be forever changing.

There is no ultimate arrival in terms of personal growth. As soon as we become aware of one thing, there is another thing to become aware of. We will be arriving at becoming until our last breath.

Nature is a perfect model of exponential growth. Picture a field of green grass, a tree full of new spring leaves. The harvest of our spirit is at hand. We can make the harvest more bountiful by inviting ourselves to make a change. Go into your control room and look at the many emotional switches that are there. How did they get there? Who put them there?

I am at the point that I often think, *Does it even matter anymore?* No. What matters is that I am at the control room's door and I have walked into the master control room. I see it running me and I can disengage the switches that no longer serve who I am now. I can give myself new messages and have new emotional responses to circumstances in my life. There is no perfect response and there is no ultimate response. There is only flexible adjustment to continual growth.

"What do you believe in?" "What do you mean?" "Can you embrace the universe?" "Well, when you can embrace the universe, come to me and ask me what I believe in and I will tell you that I believe in that and more. There is always more."

The more of you will be at your door in a dream, a thought, when you are driving your car! "Hello, buddy, what's up?" You may not have an easy answer to that, but you will have fun thinking about it. What could you do if you changed your mind about yourself and your life? You would change your life! Pretty cool!

When you think of *Return to the Soul of Your Child* and also "Soul of a Child," think of messages that surround a young child. There are thousands of messages that they receive in the course of their lifetime. There is an imprint that is made from this format of words that will guide life's decisions for the rest of their lives. It may take a person into adulthood. It may take that long for a person to question these formats or a person may never question, but simply accept them as who they are. There are many roads that are not taken because of mental formatting. The key to life is reflection and reassessment. We are lucky if we have had the opportunity to do this. Word upon word format our lives. Give your life some new words! You decide what messages you wish to carry and live out!

Start with small things and move to bigger issues in your life. You are the scriptwriter and it is your choice to change or not to change. It is your adventure of self. If you have just become aware of the power of your words, the wonderful resilience of children leads them to quickly absorb new words and they flow easily into rerouted formats. Adults have more ingrained formats and it takes more effort to consciously reset these formats. The try-again theme is helpful. How do we motivate ourselves and others? The power of our words. Your mind is your tool for living this life. Employ it! Enjoy it! As more people become aware of this, more changes will begin to take place for many people.

Returning to the idea of personal formats, consider looking at your mindset. What has put it into place? Do you monitor it? Are you gaining self-mastery over your personal mindset? This is where your work can begin.

You may or may not have children you are having an influence over, but you are in fact influencing yourself with every word you think and speak. This is a good place to start. The adventure will begin when you track your threads of formatting and they lead you to a source. Then you have to decide how to reformat and release this old imprint from the past. How fun for you! This is not me at this time and so delete it! Input a new desired format! I am worth it and yes, I can! So your adventure begins and ends with words that surround you. Words start your day and words end your day. You are returning to the soul of your child and resetting formats by your own decision. You will reset your life's course and help anyone else that you share your life with!

Each person's journey is unique and surrounded by their own special circumstances. Getting over yourself and getting over everyone else will allow you to stand free of judgment. The adventure is deciding on the new format and how it may best serve your life at the present time. Life is moment to moment and so it will change as needed. Meet and greet your gifts and be aware that they may have been trying to get your attention your entire life.

If you pursue a new interest and it is an enrichment, great! It will make your heart happier! What we do as an extended interest does not have to serve a monetary purpose. It just might be something we do that makes our heart happy! Things that make our face smile and our heart happy are good! Once you have gained a level of awareness of one thing, you will become aware of another thing. You will never be done growing. You are never done becoming who you are. Life is a forever journey!

If we can remember that we are formatted with the language that surrounds us, we will become more mindful in our use and application of language in the varying relationships that we are in. As you discover the great adventure of your own consciousness, you will start to enjoy a new sense of self and experience new energy in your life. The gift of self-mastery is freedom from self-limitation. We limit ourselves with our preconceived ideas of who we think we are.

Let your messages to yourself and others be supportive of the growth of consciousness and expansion of their abilities. There are many other people who have uncultivated gifts of spirit. If you feel a nudge to try something new, try it! Experience it and don't judge your first attempts to do something new. If you are doing something new and having fun, enjoy the experience and allow yourself to enjoy it. Do not measure it in a serious way. Fun and joy free our energy in life and make us more available for other experiences.

As your personal expansion continues, you will experience more and more of yourself. It is personally empowering to find your value as a human being and cultivate it and see it grow. It is also rewarding to know that you are trying to take a conscious position in how your words affect people that you share your life with. Activate your unlimited self with reflection, reformatting, and awareness.

We are scriptwriters after all. We hear our spirit call us to a new day. Our lives continue to unfold, the greatest story ever told. We find our way there. Life's sweet, dark mystery is revealed as light and shadow in a field. We stand there. As we stand in the field of life and become aware of the contrast, we can decide what we want to experience and what we want more of. Then, we work on and shift our patterns and activate the patterns and release old formats we no longer want to experience.

Dynamic supportive language will help you create the new reality that you picture in your mind. Use your mental pictures to help you build a new ocean of words that flows around you and the ones you share your life with each day. You can forge a new identity built on positive formatting! You will be looking at your formatting and redesigning it to suit who you are. It should give you relief to know that we are all works in progress and that there will always be something else to consider. The words that surround you and others are embedded in them as their personal truth. Decisions are made based on these personal truths.

Just because a person of influence says that you are this or you are that does not make that particular observation of you accurate. It is simply their perception of their view of you. Take what everyone says with a grain of salt. Evaluate their opinion and then build your own assessment based on what you know to be true. Everything requires time and effort. To build a new personal truth will give you a scaffold upon which you can springboard to new life experiences.

Life Is a Healing Journey

Life is a healing journey. After our formatting is set, we replay the frequency in our daily lives. We set up similar experiences in various venues of life. As we become aware of our part in the creation of our lives with words, we can set ourselves free from the conscripts of those experiences or sets of formats. As we face our present self with our active present formats, we can review our acquisition of them. They have been layered over time and years of living. Key players in our lives have helped us acquire them. If you observe yourself doing and saying things in a repetitive way and you don't like what you see yourself doing or saying—stop! Reflect, reassess, and begin the process of reformatting yourself. If you think of a control center with a master switchboard and you are the controller of the switch—you can start to enter your switchboard room with authority. As you start to react in a preconditioned way, you can stop and think, *I am turning that switch off now*. Break the connection with that frequency. Reroute your personal energy.

One of the most challenging personal patterns that I work on to reroute is using food as a response to stress. There are many ways to become self-aware. It is a personal choice how we become aware of our formatting. If your life's stressors activate a behavior response that you know is counterproductive to healthy living, assess it—look at it and find a way that works for you to reformat your personal response to stress. If your conditioned loop keeps looping around and you return to the same behavior, then try to create a mental picture of your master panel of switches. Enter the control room and throw off the switch that has been activated by life stressors. You insert the desired pattern of behavior that you want to create.

Each of us is who we are based upon our life's conditioning. My earlier life's conditional patterns were not particularly supportive of gifts that my later life revealed. These gifts lie dormant within the person and the potentiality is there. Everyone has dormant potential that has not been triggered. It may remain dormant depending upon the lifetime of the individual.

We only have to remove the mental programming of our past and insert formats of our own choosing. As I continued to move into higher education and became immersed in academics, I felt the great desire to help others become aware of their hidden gifts. My musical gift was loud and persistent. Check out my website, Graceful Road Music.com.

The cds of music on my website are a testimony to this gift. I am grateful to this gift for pointing out the discrepancies between what I could do with music and what I had been told that I could do as a very young person. I was told I have no musical ability. "You can't carry a tune in a basket but your voice is loud. You have no musical ability."

I did not pick up a guitar until my mid to late twenties. The river of tone flowed into my mind and brought great joy to my life. It was something that I did in-between wash loads and my small children's naps.

I had my songs scored and copyrighted. I shared them whenever I could. They were well received. I still had a hard time reconciling what I had been told so emphatically as a young person: "Take up typing and shorthand." "You have no musical ability." I believed the message and, until the urge to play guitar in my twenties, had no desire to pursue music.

I learned to read music in between wash loads. I ended up teaching at a local music store for nineteen years. I also taught guitar at a junior college for eleven years. I produced and marketed a book called *The Unicorn's Gift*. That effort put me on the map as a musician and a music teacher. Teaching music showed me that I enjoyed teaching people. I became a classroom teacher at the age of fifty and taught until I was sixty-two. I obtained a master's degree in education at the age of sixty. My master's work was about self-efficacy and the support of it in the public school classroom.

Self-Efficacy

Self-efficacy is a person's belief based on actual skill, of one's ability to do a task. There is a way of creating support for people's willingness to try something new, to allow them to try and grow in a skill. I knew this is something I wanted to share with many people because of my own struggles in following the call of my gift. Hey, hello there! Anybody home! That is my invitation to the reader! Look into your heart. Look into your mind and see what is trying to get your attention. Each gift is different. Each experience is different. Believe me when I tell you that if your gift decides to call you, it will get your attention! I strongly suspect that there are many unclaimed gifts of spirit that would love to manifest into people's lives. For starters, let your happiness out! Have fun! Play! I am never so happy as when I am singing and I only like to sing my songs!

I know as the years went by, I accepted my gift, and so did my family. Grudgingly at first, and then they were resigned to it that I was a musician. So why did I bother to tell you this story? Because there is someone out there who will respond to it. They will think about it and then bump, their gift will say hello! Hey! Anybody home?

Invite your unlimited self out to play and say hello to it. Be willing to evaluate the things that you think are a given about yourself and analyze them and determine if your continued improvement as a soul and the continued improvement of any children in your life are worth your time. Yes! We are worthy of another look! Don't take face value what you believe to be your truths! What does your heart resonate to? What does your mind resonate to?

Build new responses to life by supporting your soul with beautiful supportive language and also the souls of children to whom you are connected. Vygotsky's legacy talks about mediated language. When we change our formatting, we are mediating our personal formats. We can have a more positive response to life.

There is science behind language mediation. As individuals, you can change the language that surrounds your mind and your heart. This will have an effect on the lives of people who are part of your life experience. Leve Vygotsky viewed the teacher as "the agent [who] guides the child's thinking." When we reset our data, we are guiding our living with new words.

As our personal self-efficacy improves, our lives improve. Today, it is simply not possible to explain phenomena such as human motivation, learning self-regulation, and accomplishment without discussing the role played by self-efficacy beliefs" (Pajares: 2006, p. ix.). Self-efficacy is rooted in the core belief that one has the power to effect changes by ones actions" (Pajares and Banduta: 2006, p.3). We internalize ways of thinking from the way we are talked to over time. The longer we have lived our lives, the more extensive our input. We have a lot of data on file that we carry as our truth. When we become the mediator of our own personal programs-formatting, we can change our lives! It is empowering to know that! Set your expectations high enough to get you to stretch into new growth.

Why wouldn't a person want to live a more positive, vigorous life experience? Change your mind, change your life. When you analyze your own personal programs, you give yourself the power to change how you live your life! Non-judgmental growth is the goal. Use your ocean of words to support your life in a flowing and growing way.

Find ways to guide yourself to more positive choices in your life, as well as the young ones whose lives you touch with your words. If old patterns return, gently release them and replace them with the patterns you want in place for your behaviors that you want to make a part of your life. Invite change with gentle restatement of the desired change that will help it to replace the pattern you want to change. Our work is never done. We need to review, evaluate, and keep on working on things we want to improve. The soul of a child and our soul will benefit from a change of language. How do you speak to yourself and others? Do you want to maintain this in life or do you want to experience an improved version of your life experience? The power is in your words and you are the one who speaks them. You are the one who thinks your thoughts!

If we stop to think about one another and the lives we are sharing, we are all just bundled programmed connections of experiences! Our group of conditioned response responds to another person's conditioned responses. We can try to wake up and become more aware of the part we play in our daily life transactions. That growing awareness will change our lives and the lives of those around us!

Day to Day
Hour to Hour
Within each is a power
To grow out and beyond where they are
All the growth is within
It is there we begin to
Explore and expand
Who we are!

One thing I know for sure
The darkness follows every day time.
Another thing for sure
We're all born
We all die

Another thing for sure
Each life's a seed planted in springtime
Every day there's growth
Reaching high!

My life's gift has given rise to many questions. The most important question I can ask the reader is, "Are you on the lookout for your gifts of life?" They are there! Listen for them, look for them. Find them, cultivate them, and if the messages that you received in life have not prepared you to know that they are there, enjoy the mystery of your life as it unfolds. The opportunity to grow and encourage others to grow is the purpose of this book. In my sixty-four years of living, I have observed that you can grow past old formats and into new ones. You can acquire new direction and go towards new vistas of self. The old horizon has left and a new one stretches out in front of us. We can meet and greet our gifts and cultivate them. Everything is one step at a time.

Stepping out of judgment leaves us free to grow. People have been formatted by the window of time they were born into and the cultures that supported their growth. They are the result of their life experiences. None of us is free from these family, cultural formats. Have compassion for the ones who gave you your formats because they also were formatted by their lives. Hand to hand, heart to heart, reach out and help each other.

Change is a part of nature and we are part of nature. Change is good. Whenever you feel an old format, go back to your master control room, enter the room, and look at your switchboard. You work the switches. Make the choice that you want to make in terms of your actions and reactions. Turn off the old switch and turn on a new one that you want to activate. This is the beginning of self-mastery.

When I was making friends with my musical gift, I did wonder about what might have happened if there had been a different response to me as a person growing up. What might have I done with my "gift"? The best part of this story is that I am sharing the possibility that there is a multitude of other people with sleeping gifts! Heads up! You may have a gift that you don't even know about. Learn to talk to yourself and others in a way that will allow you to go forward in your life in a joyful way so that you will want to try new things and have fun!

As you reflect on your living, you can come to know you made as many positive changes in your life that you could and tried to be a positive influence in the lives of the people you shared your experience with. That's enough to give you peace. You can't change anyone's mind but your own. All the growth is within you and you are free to make changes or not. Become aware of your personal formats and change the ones that no longer serve you. Choose your words carefully and know that they are a force for good in the world. Meet and greet your unlimited self and have fun! Your consciousness is an adventure and as you explore and expand, it will manifest more of your potential. Grow, grow, and grow! Like the trees in spring!

Intellect which separates we need a heart to join
Forces in the living being
For their life's sojourn.
Mind without a loving heart
Heart without a mind
Ah the crises these have formed
Tragedies entwined.

Separate these forces stand
To break and to destroy
But enjoined they create
A powerful alloy

So these forces do enjoin and
You'll surely stand
To put together pieces
Where havoc's played its hand.

Intellect that separates
We need a heart to join
Forces in the living being
For their life's sojourn.

The intellect and the heart can work together. As science and holistic methods become aware of each other, it will be seen that heart wisdom has value as well as mind or intellect value. The two together can do amazing things. This life has been a journey of the mind and heart. The emotions or heart alone need the balance of intellect and then more dynamic life experiences can begin to be lived. Left brain, right brain, one benefits the other!

There are different ways of thinking that can achieve similar outcomes. Opening our minds to our possibilities can change lives. We all have to do our own work, or own growth. That is the adventure of each life. How can we bring into play people's willingness to try new things? We support their efforts. We support their efforts with words that lead them to the increased effort that builds the necessary skill trying to be cultivated. If it is a traditional classroom, teaching music, whatever the discipline, the trying is what is going to build the next level of skill. If the teacher, guide, or parent can become aware of the power of guiding words, the respective student will be more willing to extend the effort to try whatever the task at hand is.

The greatest calling that all of us has is to open our minds to the myriads of possibilities that we have in front of us to achieve. It is all a step at a time. Open our minds and hearts to our possibilities and use supportive language that gives a scaffold of willingness to try new tasks. This can help lead students in whatever discipline to increased effort and eventually to increased skill level in the area being developed. Try again is not a wasted thought. Try again is necessary for growth.

The mind's ability to comprehend that there is value to the attempt is enough to activate the student's willingness to try the task. This is why it is important to stress the positive value of the person and their efforts to attempt or try the task. Learning how to create mediated language in your life will help whatever areas of your life that you are trying to improve. Supportive language mediation is a critical component to student success if you are a teacher and personal success if you are applying it to your own personal life. A supportive learning or living environment and an invitation to try things with supportive language will build the necessary bridge to increased effort. Increased effort will eventually build whatever new life skills you or someone that you influence is trying to acquire!

Going back to the idea that the myriads of possibilities are available to each and every soul on the planet: Opening the mind will enable people to be willing to try new things that they have never tried before. Everyone's journey is different. The lessons of each life are different. Different paths of life experience lead us to growth. If we find a teacher who can invite us to open our minds and try that is the first step. It is each person's adventure to cultivate their experiences and go forward in their life finding their unique service. Service in life usually is confined to traditional assigned roles in human relationships. Husband, wife, parents, grandparents, children, teachers, ministers, administrators, doctors, lawyers—we are all in service to one another.

People try to define themselves predicated upon the life message that they have received and the experiences they have had. When people can jump-start their growth is when they can step outside of the definition of who they think they are and grow into new possibilities of expression in their individual lives. There is a greater expansion of human consciousness right now. It is important for all of us to step out of our preconceived ideas of who we think we are and cultivate new adventures. This, again for all of us, is a step at a time. One step and then another is all any of us have.

Irregardless of where we are in life, we are in service to one another. Our service does not depend upon a vocation. It depends upon who we are born to and what opportunities those circumstances provide for us to develop our potential. We all continue to learn from one another. You may see someone homeless on the street. This person is learning a life lesson and as you pass them by, you are also learning from them. Every life experience offers a life lesson to the person living it.

Again, not to be redundant but to emphasize the ability of people to open their mind and try something that they are trying to learn will allow them to experience the more of who they are. The unlimited self is ever unfolding; we do not even consider ourselves unlimited because of life's assigned roles. We have taken on our roles within marriages, careers, jobs, hobbies. These roles help to inform us of who we think we are. There is more beyond that picture of who we think we are. There is always more.

I know that the anvil of my message is based on my experience with music. If you check out my website, http://gracefulroadmusic.com, you will see the music that I found and shared. I was told as a child that I had no musical ability and could not sing. The CDs and compositions are created by me, this unmusical person! These early life messages precluded me touching an instrument until my middle twenties. Music was my hobby. I strummed my first guitar in-between my babies' naps! I found and cultivated music. I know that my experience is not unique. I know that there are many uncultivated gifts in many, many other people. I bumped into my "gift". I had a wonderful time with it and have enjoyed sharing and singing my songs for many years. I know based upon my education and experience as a public school teacher that we respond to the messages that we receive. My master's work, *Support of Student Self-Efficacy in the Public School Classroom*, can be accessed in the library archives of California State University of Monterey Bay. It is available to anyone who wants to access the study. I would like to encourage educators and parents and anyone who works with a young clientele to look at the study. We are

40

formatted by the language that surrounds us. The study is supported by academic work. Think about it! You might find something in it that may be of service to you!

To empower yourself and everyone who you come in contact with become aware of the influence of language. The language that you use every day is a structure of living that binds each breath you take to the next breath. Language connects life and the life of the soul. Each soul is impacted by it. We can free our potential and the potential of others by gaining an awareness of this basic but transformational fact. The power of language was discovered by Leve Vygotsky. His work was cutting edge in the 1930s and is coming into play now. More and more educators are becoming aware of the powerful work that this scholar left behind for people to discover and use today. Reference to his work can be found in my master's work previously mentioned.

Words make life happen. Positive words, guiding words make a difference to everyone in every setting of life. Have you ever been in line at the grocery store and had a small mishap happen? For example, let's say there is a small child trying to help his or her mother put a jar of food in the basket. The jar slips from the small child's hand and breaks on the floor. The mother is aggravated, the line stiffens, the child is ready to be reprimanded, but then someone in the line makes the simple comment, "It could have happened to anyone." The mother sighs a sigh of relief, the lines relaxes. A store clerk comes up with a mop and life flows on. The child had an accident that could have happened to anyone of us. Oh, well, we clean it up and move on. Soft words, sigh of relief, and life goes on. That's how it works. Just simple words in simple life transactions can build a bridge of growth and hope for every one of us. We all need kind words and gentle guidance to the next step. The gift of our words is what we can give to one another. A breath at a time and a word at a time. Find our gifts and cultivate them. Share your gifts and if they give you joy in a hobby, enjoy them! Joy leads us to more joy. Smiles lead us to more smiles.

Another thing to be aware of is that we all have different levels of understanding of the power of our words. Some folks will not think that there is any impact on their lives or anyone's life just because of words. You can try and observe; if you choose all of your words to be supportive and gentle in one day, what kind of day would you have? Try it! See what happens! It could begin to create a new adventure for you. A day full of kind, supportive words! Would it soften a business transaction, a communication with a child in your life? It won't cost you anything and you might be amazed at the change in the energy of yourself and everyone else that you are connected to.

Your life's journey is going to take you many places. You will have countless personal transactions in the course of your life—from childhood into young adulthood and into later life. Consider the power of your words. Wherever you are in your life, you can start right now. Some of us become aware at an earlier age and can make use of this information sooner. It is never too late to become aware of the power of your words. Our words are setting the vibrational frequency of our day. You are the activator of your tongue. If you become aware of that, then you can use it with a positive purpose in your life.

Your life is a canvas wherein you paint a new experience every day. Each thought, each choice, each relationship is another part of your canvas of living. You are the artist of your own life. What is on your canvas? Each day gives you a new canvas on which to paint your life experience. Look at the easel; pick up the brush (your tongue), and go! There you are! If you don't like what you see, set a new intention and paint again. As long as we breathe, we are the artist. When one set of circumstances changes, flow with it. Pick up your brush and set your intention for whatever you would like to see on the canvas of your life. What a deal! Use the power of your mind right now. You don't need a guru to do this. You don't need to live on a mountaintop and you don't need to look outside of yourself to do this. Just start where you are and have fun with your life!

Fun right in your kitchen, garage, backyard, place of worship, store, workplace—right where you are. Be in the moment. We only have the next moment. All of our moments add up to a lifetime. What is the story of your life? What is the song that your heart sings? Step outside of the box that you have put yourself in and reflect. Perhaps draw another box and experience that. Unlimited self, "Hello there"! People have the potential to imagine themselves as different from what they are. Remember when you were six years old and you wanted to be ten years old? It happened. Then you wanted to be fifteen or sixteen years old because then you could wear lipstick on Sundays? Well, you keep changing and becoming. Surprise yourself by inviting out your new self to play!

The next step in the adventure is that once you have opened your mind to the possibility that you have things to do that you have never done, you allow yourself to cultivate that interest. You are never done with this process. One thing and then another. We set our own limits for the most part. Circumstances can impact a life's journey that has an effect on the direction, but we can reroute and continue on. That is true for all of us. There is not only one path to who we are. This is a very freeing thought. There is not just one path to who we are. We go on many adventures in the course of our life time. As we become aware, we actively participate in the creation of our lives. We develop a level of mindfulness that makes our experiences truly our own. See the blank paper, pick up the pen, you are the scriptwriter. What is the script that you are writing?

We are scriptwriters after all
We hear our spirit call us to a new day!
Our lives continue to unfold!
The greatest stories ever told!
We find our way there.
We grow in spirit, body, mind
We leave the past behind.
Our stories flowing
Life's sweet dark mystery is revealed
As light and shadow in a field.
We stand there.

Use your language to guide young people in your life to more growth. If you create mediated language in your own life with those you have influence over, you can have a positive effect on their growth. Feel free to use the research of my master's study previously mentioned! It can be a useful tool in becoming aware of this language effect! Feel free to create your own language scaffold for whatever purposes that you may have in various areas of service in your life.

Each strand of *The Active Learner Mediated Scaffold* that I will include with this book is supported by a scholarly study.

Feel free to use the scaffold, as I am the author of this work. It is my intention to share it with as many educators and mothers and fathers as I can. Anyone in service to child can make use of this work. You can change the way you say things. Make it work for the field of service that you are working in. Check out the study *Support of Student Self-Efficacy in the Public School Classroom* and see the difference it made in the lives of California School Children for the two years that it was in use. It works!

In short, the language mediation scaffold guides student effort. This supports student self-efficacy. Anyone using a positive language scaffold can have a positive effect on the environment one is in service. Your environment may be a kitchen with small children running around, or a business setting that is touching many lives. Your setting may be a formal classroom that touches many minds and hearts. It is a useful tool. It is available. Use it!

This is just one idea in terms of a language scaffold of positive supporting thoughts. People could create their own for their own children or their own classrooms. Lev Vygotsky's work is inspiring and will give many other educators and parents new ideas to work with. Supportive words give power to a person's direction. It also gives a person permission to try. That has to be emphasized over and over again. It is the trying that will lead to new growth. Very few of us will succeed on the first attempt we try a new skill. Young and old and in-between will need to try more than once to build a new skill.

If you stop and think about all the human transactions that you have in a week, a month and a year, what impact could you make on your life if you really started to create language that comes out of your mouth mindfully? Hmmm? That is an interesting proposition. First, try it for an hour, then a day, then a week, then a month, and then a year! What is the outcome? Journal and track your progress with your own powerful language. The power of your mind and your tongue. You each have your own personal belief system, religions, and points of focus to apply this to. Change your mind—change your life. The power is yours to become aware of. One thought leads us to another thought and another action. We can transform our lives with the power of our mind.

Our words and thoughts are ours to craft our lives with. As we become aware of the power of our words and thoughts, we can begin to transform our life experiences to reflect more of who we really are. Life is an inviting adventure. Now is our moment! Now is our time!

Now is the time to claim the power of your mind, your words, and your heart. Now is the time to enter your mental garden and become aware of what is there waiting for your to put into action. You can invite yourself to experience yourself in a new way! You will begin to experience yourself in an unlimited way! It doesn't cost you anything to try or to think about it. If we tend to our lives like we tend a garden, there might begin to be a different relationship with our thoughts and our words. In a garden, weeds are pulled and plants maintained with water. The same goes for our mental and physical bodies.

The more mindfully we tend to our minds, hearts, and bodies, the better the outcome of our life experience. It is easy to be dismissive of our physical and emotional needs. If you are on a fast-moving trolley of earning a living, caring for a young family or an old family stop, take a few minutes a day to put your inner life in order. Claim your inherent rights to be more in your life by becoming aware of the part you play in the life you are living.

Your words, thoughts, and emotions form the experience you are having as a person. Help others experience more of themselves by nurturing them with words that support them. Use words that make them willing to try to do whatever tasks are there for them to do. When we think of the soul of a child, we also need to remember that once, we were a child and we were starting our journey. Even if the words that surrounded us did not make it easy for us to access our growth as a developing soul, we are who we are because of the sum total of all of our experiences. When you remember to speak to others with supportive words, you are also speaking to yourself. What you do for others, you are also indirectly doing for yourself. You will start to remove barriers placed there by inadvertent well-meaning messengers of your life. Perceived limitations will melt away and the past will no longer be in effect as your life is empowered with your newly energized words. You not only make the world more accessible for those who are part of your life, but yourself as well.

It can set you free to know that you are not bound to succeed or fail. You are only bound to learn and grow. Did you learn anything on your journey? Did you grow and did you manage to help someone else along the way? Look around you and see the world with new eyes. Notice simple gifts of daily life like a child's smile, a bird soaring, a bird's song, a flower blooming. Pause, breathe, and notice. As you become more present in your living, your words will flow more naturally into support mode. The experience of the people whom you share your life with will change and those around you will also be affected by the words that you use with them.

There is no beginning or end to personal growth. You are in this life as long as you are in this life! You are an active player as long as you are here! Have fun with your life canvas and have a good time creating new pictures every day! If you review today's experiences and you don't like what you see, paint a new picture the next day. You are the artist of your own life. You are the author of your life's script. If you don't like the story that you have been living, pick up a piece of blank paper and a pen and write the story the way you want to see it happen. Live it, feel it, breathe it in!

Keep in mind that your message or scaffold of words will be accessed in different ways by different people. Each person will have each own way of processing what you have told him or her. Do not take it personally if you have a particular outcome in mind and something else occurs! Share you message and the response is what it is. You have control over yourself and your own progress, but you are not in charge of anyone else's growth. Just do your best to share your message.

People respond differently depending on what they have previously experienced and the stage of life that they are in. There may be influences in their lives that you have no control over. If you can keep that in mind, you will be at peace with whatever the outcome is of your life's adventure. It is an adventure for everyone. Travel your road with assurance that you will keep growing and changing no matter what. We are in a continual process of assimilation and change.

We are never done becoming who we are. You will never have arrived at a final destination.

What is in the garden of your spirit? Kind words that you never spoke? Are there songs that you never took the time to write? Is there a book or two that was never written and shared? Visit your inner garden from time to time and spend time there. You can do it in prayer or meditation. You can do it in your own way. Spend time there. As you learn to go into your own inner garden, you will find more of your unlimited self emerging. You will become more aware of yourself.

When you are working with your new supportive language scaffold and empowering your life, there may be times when you are more aware of it than others. Some days as you reflect, you may want to redo the day in your mind and as a new day unfolds, you want to put into play what you would have liked to see in your personal transactions with other people in your daily life. The most invigorating thing about this awareness is that it is unique with each person and you will work with it in terms that you can apply to your own life.

Consider the language that you have the power to create with your unlimited mind. Our minds are more powerful than any computer and we don't use much of them. Harness your power to change your life. Change your life according to the canvas that you want to paint. New day, new canvas, new picture! Create! Enjoy! Become! Manifest! Transform!

Taking your life's journey to new dimensions is an opportunity that is worth taking. We can experience new dimensions of self if we expand our mental horizons to embrace new ideas and new ways of thinking, speaking, and being. Think of this as an opportunity to experience more of yourself and your life. Such a simple thing as words: How do you talk to people? How do they talk to you? Do you like the way you talk to people and do you like the way people talk to you. Talk, talk, talk, and talk to them. Where do your words take you and where do their words take you? Some of us are born into life experiences where we were supported by loving, guiding language. Others had experiences that did not provide as secure a foothold into personal growth. No matter. We continue to grow into who we are and we are all part of the divine, whatever your personal reference. Our

47

potential is exponential and we continue to grow whatever our ages and whatever our experiences. Our experiences have led us to become who we are, and that is subject to change on a moment to moment basis. When we become aware of the mechanisms of change, we can employ them to build a better scaffold for our life experience.

As I look back at the window of time and the culture that I was born to, a lot of people were like me. The new me is a lot more fun and a lot less limited! Becoming the new me is now an ongoing adventure. My service as a classroom teacher is over, but my message is still clear and serves a purpose. The power of our words changes our lives. What kind of messages do you want in your personal database? Hmmm? You get to do the reformatting! Fun! Okay, let's see. Start with small things and then work on things that you consider to be more challenging. We can reformat ourselves by going into our mental control room, looking at our switches. Turn off any switch that you no longer want guiding your life and reformat your control room with switches that you do want guiding your life. A breakthrough for me recently was to get over myself and get over everyone else and stand out of judgment. We judge ourselves and others and it uses our personal energy. The best part of being the place I am in right now is that the past doesn't matter to me. It was my springboard to who I am now. When words that are unsupportive of you are flowing around you, don't absorb them. Try and think of the words that you want to maintain yourself with and others and put them out into your life experience. Even these unsupportive words can help us become aware of who we are. They don't feel right. They don't feel like us.

Use this as an opportunity to think and say words that you want to become a part of your life experience. Your words help to define who you want to be. You decide what those words are going to be and you make them happen in your life. Sometimes, we are the formatters and sometimes we are the ones receiving the formats!

Unlimited beings on a road of light!
Open your beautiful minds and soar!
Unlimited beings on a road of light!
Remember life's an open door!

Support of Student Self-Efficacy in the Public School Classroom

Mary O. Lesher M.A.E.
Copyright, ©, 2008

The following master's work is what the book *Return to the Soul of Your Child* was based on. It is available for parents, educators, and other lay persons to read and share. I hope that you find its content helpful and inspiring to your own work in your own lives.

Support of Student Self-Efficacy in the Public School Classroom

Action Thesis Submitted in Partial Fulfillment of the Requirements
For the Degree of Master of Arts in Education

California State University at Monterey Bay
Fall 2008

Mary O. Lesher
Approved by:

Dr. Nicholas Meier

Dr. Bill Jones

i

Acknowledgements

I would like to thank my advisor Dr. Nicholas Meier for his support of this master's project as well as Dr. Terry Arambula-Greenfield. I would also like to thank my mentor Dr. Lucindi Mooney for her belief in my becoming a teacher and her steadfast encouragement of my goals. I would also like to thank my school site Elkhorn Elementary School for the opportunity to develop this action research project there and to be of service as an elementary school teacher. A special thanks to friends and family who supported my work through the loss of my parents and would not allow me to give up. Deepest thanks to all of you.

Abstract

This action thesis project is submitted in partial fulfillment of the requirements for the Master of Arts in Education degree at California State University, Monterey Bay. This project is "Support of Student Self-Efficacy in the Public School Classroom."

This action research project is an analysis of my practice as a classroom teacher with the focus being on the support of self-efficacy of students in the elementary school classroom setting. The daily analysis of my practice in the elementary classroom revealed to me what I was doing to support student self-efficacy during lessons. The analysis also focused on the development of classroom management that reinforced student willingness to try academic tasks.

The two-hour language arts lesson that was analyzed on a daily basis revealed to me that the language that a teacher uses in the classroom can enable students to focus and try to perform academic tasks. This action research project made me aware of the impact that a classroom teacher can have on encouraging students to be active learners.

The *Active Learner Mediated Language Scaffold* resulted from the findings of this action research project. The *Active Learner Mediated Language Scaffold* is supported by scholarly studies. The *Active Learner Mediated Language Scaffold* is presently in use in elementary classrooms in this area. The findings of this study suggest that the *Active Learner Mediated Language Scaffold* supports student self-efficacy.

Table of Contents

Chapter 1

This action thesis is created for the use of teachers or anyone who may have an interest in self-efficacy in their work setting. "Self-efficacy is rooted in the core belief that one has the power to effect changes by ones actions" (Pajares & Bandura, 2006, p.3). "Self-efficacy refers to the confidence of a person in their capabilities to complete a given task successfully" (Narciss, 2004, p.4). Analysis of my practice is focused on the support of self-efficacy in the public school classroom. "Self-efficacy is widely acknowledged as one of the most important developments in the history of psychology. Today, it is simply not possible to explain phenomena such as human motivation, learning, self-regulation and accomplishment without discussing the role played by self-efficacy beliefs" (Pajares, 2006, p.ix). There are many current studies that indicate that self-efficacy plays a role in student success. A Korean study notes that self-efficacy in students "fluctuated significantly around examinations" (Bong, 2005, p.l) and an international study found self-efficacy to have an impact on children's "academic self-regulatory efficacy" (Pastorelli, 2001, p.12). Self-efficacy is important to consider in the academic setting because it is another way to support student success.

Overview of Problem and Purpose

The purpose of this action research project was for me to analyze my teaching practice in terms of the support of student self-efficacy in the public school classroom. I wanted to assess my support of this important psychological construct within my daily practice. This action research project gave me the opportunity to scrutinize and evaluate my daily practice and improve it as the project progressed.

Research Question

My overall research question was as follows: How did my teaching support student self-efficacy? Within this main question, I focused more specifically on what ways my practice supported student self-efficacy thr006Fugh the following mechanisms:

- Lev Vygotsky's language mediation (Gredler & Shields, 2008).
- Feedback opportunities (Narciss, 2004).
- Teacher expectations (Rubie-Davis, 2006).
- Goal setting (Page-Voth, 1999).
- Support of student culture (Gillard, Moore & Lemieux, 2008).

Since self-efficacy is "rooted in the core belief that one has the power to effect changes by ones actions" (Pajares & Bandura, 2006, p.3), how does my practice support student self-efficacy in the public school classroom?

Personal History

In my eleven years as a classroom teacher, nineteen years as a music teacher in Salinas, California, eleven of which were at Hartnell College as a staff instructor, many years of business experience in banking, thirty years co-owner of a family business in Seaside, California and a parent of two grown children, I have always been interested in human potential. My interest in human potential has grown over time. My service in the elementary classroom in the public school setting has made me aware students respond to positive reinforcement. A particular incident that brought the issue of student selfefficacy to my attention was the following comment written by a student of mine a few years back: "I thought I wasn't going to be a wonderful person then my teacher told me I am the future. I believed her and felt better for myself." This made me feel like the experience that this student had within my classroom was a positive one. I wanted to continue to cultivate a practice that would allow other students to have a similar experience. I wanted to extend the experience to all of my students.

Definition of Terms

Self-efficacy: In this study the changes were focused on student's being willing to try academic tasks in an elementary classroom. "Self-efficacy is rooted in the core belief that one has the power to effect changes by ones actions" (Pajares & Bandura, 2006, p.3). "Self-efficacy refers to the confidence of a person in their capabilities to complete a given task successfully" (Narciss, 2004, pA).

Feedback opportunities: When a teacher gives students feedback on their work it allows them to see what they need to do to either maintain their effort or to redirect their efforts in terms of academic performance. "The term informative tutoringfeedback (ITF) refers to feedback types providing strategically useful information that guides the learner toward successful task completion" (Narciss, 2004, p.3).

Goal setting: Goal setting is when a desired outcome is outlined and modeled for students. Goal setting is an important strategy in elementary classroom settings. When behavior and performance goals are set, students have a scaffold that suggests a course of academic action that may lead them to increased academic performance. Academic performance in the classroom is "a goal directed activity" "Specific goals" (p.3) that allow students to learn with "a directional function" (Page-Voth, 1999, pA) assist in student academic performance (Page-Voth, 1999).

Active Learner: An active learner is a student that is practicing strands of the Active Learner Mediated Language Scaffold, and who is taking an active role in their learning during lessons. Active Learner was a term that came to my attention in the de Haan study which was a study about action learning (de Haan, 2006). This study was a study about adult learning but the term could be applied to learning action in an elementary classroom.

Parameters of Study

The *Active Learner Mediated Language Scaffold* that emerged during this action research project resulted in the development and design of a helpful classroom tool created to support student's self-efficacy. Its design supports specific classroom behaviors that allow students to focus and attempt the many academic tasks that they face every day in their elementary classroom. The use of the *Active Learner Mediated Language Scaffold* is supported by the work of Lev Vygotsky. Vygotsky viewed the teacher as "the agent that guides the child's thinking" (Gredler & Shields, p. 89). The daily use of the *Active Learner Mediated Language Scaffold* at the beginning and during the day's lessons provides students with a set of behaviors that guide their efforts in their academic tasks. New teachers that are just learning how to manage their classrooms may find the use of the Active Learner Mediated Language Scaffold helpful to their practice. Experienced teachers may find it helpful in that it is a slightly different approach than they may have been using, (Gredler & Shields, 2008; Narciss, 2004; Page-Voth, 1999; Rubie-Davis, 2006).

Overview of Project

Chapter one includes statement of purpose, introduction to the issue, overview of the problem and purpose, research question, personal history, and definition of terms. Chapter two is the literature review that aligns the study, its problem, purpose and research question within the academic literature. The third chapter explains the qualitative research design that was used for this action research project. The fourth chapter reveals the results and findings of this study. The fifth chapter presents my plan for future action of the use of the *Active Learner Mediated Language Scaffold*.

Chapter 2
Literature Review

In this section, I will be reviewing the literature that informs my research question how did my teaching support student self-efficacy? I will look first at the literature that identifies and defines self-efficacy. I will then discuss the literature that explains Vygotsky's perspective of the teacher in the classroom. In addition, I will discuss research that pertains to feedback opportunities, teacher expectations and goal setting. Finally, I will conclude with research that pertains to student culture.

"Self-efficacy is widely acknowledged as one of the most important developments in the history of psychology. Today it is simply not possible to explain phenomena such as human motivation, learning, self-regulation and accomplishment without discussing the role played by self-efficacy beliefs" (Pajares, 2006, p.ix). Self-efficacy is rooted in the core belief that one has the power to effect changes by ones actions" (Pajares & Bandura, 2006, p.3). Research indicates that the impact that self-efficacy has on student performance is significant. Self-efficacy is a psychological construct that everyone has and that everyone is effected by. It is an internal process that is directed from within the mind (Pastorelli, 2001; Scholz, Guiterrez, Sud, & Schwarzer, 2002). What might assist connection with individual self-efficacy? Can student self-efficacy be supported in the elementary classroom?

"Vygotsky viewed the teacher as the model from who the child internalizes ways of thinking." He viewed the teacher as "the agent that guides the child's thinking" (Gredler & Shields,2008, p.89). The teacher is the mediator of the classroom setting and uses "simple signs that manage and control one's thinking on cognitive tasks" (p.51). There are different academic mechanisms that can assist children in their thinking. One of these academic mechanisms feedback.

In a study of the relationship between teacher feedback and student self-efficacy and performance, it was found that students with low self-efficacy do not benefit from the feedback as much as students with medium or higher self-efficacy. The outcome of this study was the findings that informative tutoring feedback could benefit student progress depending on their level of self-efficacy (Narciss, 2004).

Feedback during the course of instruction mayor may not benefit student self-efficacy.

Feedback is still an important academic mechanism that may offer some support to student self-efficacy.

Teacher expectations is another academic mechanism that provides guidance to students in their academic tasks. That student self-perception in academic areas "appeared to change over the year in relation to teachers' expectations" is important and has implications for practicing teachers as well as for preservice teacher education programs (Rubie-Davies, 2006). According to research, teacher expectations are important to students.

Goal setting is an academic mechanism that helps strengthen student learning experiences. "Establishing goals that specify what will be included in a composition can have a salutatory effect on these students' writing" (Page-Voth, 1999, p.15). Goal setting is an important strategy for an educator to use to help students incorporate into their learning. When a student is given a specific goal to accomplish, it helps them to see what they need to do to succeed that goal. Goal setting helps them set into motion the action they need to take as an active participant in their learning. Goal setting can be used to increase student's productivity (Page-Voth, 1999). When students experience increased productivity, their self-efficacy may increase because "whatever factors serve as guides and motivators, they are rooted in the core belief that one has the power to effect changes by ones actions" (Pajares & Bandura, 2006, p.3).

Student culture is important to student self-efficacy. Student culture may mediate the way that the classroom is run. The culture of a student and their family has a direct effect on how they respond to academic elements presented in the classroom setting. Educators must be culturally aware of their students. It is important for an educator to be aware of "the importance of respecting and researching parent' beliefs and preferences and the need to shape the curriculum and teaching based on family values and view points" (Gillard, Moore & Lemieux, 2008, p.7). Vygotsky's perspective emphasizes that "the development of the child's thinking depends on his mastery of the social means of thinking, that is, on his mastery of speech....The child lacks the basic tools of thinking in the print language of the culture" (Gredler & Shields, p. 120). Students with non-standard English or another home language base face a particular challenge in the public school classroom. The educator in this setting must be aware of student culture and the importance of the support of that culture.

The literature that supports this study emphasizes Bandura's and Pajare's definition of self-efficacy, Vygotsky's language mediation, feedback opportunities, teacher expectations, goal setting and support of student culture. I choose this plan of action because my classroom is where I can make a difference for students. I want to determine if my practice supports the important psychological construct self-efficacy. I would like to analyze and evaluate my work in terms of continued improvement. It is also important for me to endeavor to add a study that might provide insight for other educators who have an interest in self-efficacy.

Chapter 3
Methodology and Procedures

This was a qualitative teacher action research project. The research question that was analyzed was, how did my teaching support student self-efficacy in my elementary classroom? This study was a self-study of my teaching practice at a rural elementary school.

Procedures in Detail

My basic teaching for the language arts block began at 9:00 a.m. every morning. Students would line up to enter my classroom. I would greet them at the door and ask them to come into the classroom. They would be directed by me to get out their Open Court text books and work books. The scripted, mandated lesson was followed on a daily and weekly basis as I was following a pacing guide. I adhered strictly to the pacing guide. Lessons are periodically monitored by the administration of my school. The daily language arts lessons have a vocabulary section, a comprehension component and a writing component. Most lessons took five to seven days to complete.

I alternate between direct instruction to the whole group of students to creating opportunities for peer exchange between students. There were times in my teaching that the students were doing the listening to the instruction and other times the classroom was buzzing with student peer exchanges during the language arts lesson. My teaching incorporates opportunities for visual learners to illustrate their favorite part of stories that were read by drawing a picture of it as well as writing several sentences about it. I also monitor student progress during lessons by walking around the entire room. I also monitor peer exchange to encourage students to work on the topic that was being taught. I paused to look at student work and give students feedback during the language arts lesson.

What began to be different for me during the instruction of this language arts block during this action research project is that I started to use mediated language to guide student performance.

Setting

This study took place at a rural elementary school. This school serves students from kindergarten to sixth grade. There are over six hundred students at this school. This school has been in existence for over fifty years. It has changed in demographics over time. The demographic configuration of the school is approximately 1% African American, 2% Asian, 2% Filipino, 76% Hispanic or Latino, 1% Pacific Islander, 19% White (not Hispanic) 67% economically disadvantaged, 47% English learners and 5% students with disabilities. There are about thirty three teachers with full credentials.

Participants

The participants of this study were my 4th grade students. The class that I taught for this action research project was a combination class of 3rd and 4th grade students. The flow of the classroom day is one that entails students leaving my classroom at 9:00 a.m. The third grade homeroom students leave my classroom and go to 3rd grade teachers for their reading block. Fourteen students remain from the homeroom group and an additional fifteen students come to my classroom for reading instruction. The total number of students in the two hour reading block is twenty nine. It is my instruction of these twenty nine fourth grade students during this language block that I studied. Twenty three of these students were English language learners. Seventy-nine percent of my reading class was' English language learners. Twenty-one percent were English only student

Data Collection

I created my action research data from my two-hour block of teaching the above students. I recorded as much of what I said and did during this block of instruction that I could remember every day. The notes were made at the end of the instruction when I had time to enter them. They were printed out from the classroom computer and brought to my personal computer be transcribed into observations in the evening. These daily journals resulted in one hundred fourteen pages of observations about my daily practice. These daily journal entries were coded into categories. The different categories were analyzed in regard to self-efficacy. They include:

- Feedback opportunities,
- Teacher expectations;
- Goal setting.

Student work was examined with respect to the student efforts to complete tasks. What this means is that, if students attempted to complete their class work, their attempts to complete the work was analyzed in terms of self-efficacy and not assessed quantitatively. This study was a reflection of my practice in the classroom and support of student self-efficacy in my practice. Students' classroom behaviors that were observed were:

- Students' attempts to accomplish a task or try including
- Students' responses to teacher questions,
- Students' interactions during peer exchange,
- Students' body language in the classroom as they were attempting different academic tasks.

Data Analysis

Thematic data analysis was used in this study. The analysis was primarily focused on my practice. I started to process my observation notes during my brief breaks from teaching. I would then take the notes home and transcribe them into action research observations. The notes were then coded and then analyzed for commonalities which will be examined in the findings.

Chapter 4
Results

In the beginning of this study, I did not often see students come into class prepared to learn. Self-efficacy is a person's self-belief based on actual skill of performance. I wondered if I could support student self-efficacy in a way that might motivate student effort during lessons. I often saw students come into class unfocused and scattered. Many times they were unable to focus their minds into their work. The one area of my teaching that I have freedom in is in my management of the classroom. The Active Learner Mediated Language Scaffold that is discussed in the results section was applied to this area of my practice.

The use of the Active Learner Mediated Language Scaffold was developed over the course of this project. My conceptual framework for organizing this information was to identify the mediated language with the mechanisms identified in the research question "How does my teaching support student self-efficacy?" *The Active Learner Mediated Language Scaffold* follows:

- An Active Learner sits up straight.
- An Active Learner calms down inside.
- An Active Learner opens up their mind.
- An Active Learner claims their power to learn.
- An Active Learner tries to do the learning task.
- An Active Learner knows that it is their responsibility to learn.
- Go Active Learners!
- You are the future!

My conceptual concept for organizing this information was to align the observations with the mechanisms in the research question "How did my teaching support student self-efficacy?" The mechanisms that were part of this conceptual concept were:

- Vygotsky's language mediation
- Feedback opportunities
- Teacher expectations
- Goal setting
- Support of student culture

When this action research project began on November 9, 2007, I was faced with the task of making my notes on my practice after I had taught a block of Language Arts to a group of twenty-seven learners. What I observed in my practice was that I was becoming aware of what I said to students before we began our mandated scripted lessons. As I observed students and how they worked, I tried to become aware of how I supported their self-efficacy. As I considered self-efficacy in the classroom, I tried to picture in my mind what it would be like to be a young learner. Would I have a strong sense of who I was or what I could do? I thought that a young person might like to experience their own sense of self. One thing I thought of is that personal power comes from becoming aware of it in the first place.

An Active Learner claims their power to learn

How could I set a goal that would challenge and motivate students? My first recorded use of claiming personal power began on November 9,2007. I started to say this to students before they began their work with me. *Let's claim our personal power*. During the course of this study there were twenty-five references to students claiming their power. Claiming personal power was mentioned as important to students. This use of language falls into the area of teacher expectations. The teacher expects students to become aware of themselves in their learning process. It is the individual's effort to become aware of themselves in their learning process that will enable them to move forward in terms of personal academic growth.

Students liked to grab a handful of air, pretending that it was their personal power. They liked to bring it down to their center or stomach area and put it inside of themselves. For example, on one occasion, I observed a student, not prompted by me, grab a handful of personal power, tuck it into his center and start to write furiously. Another comment made by a student was that they liked to claim their power on paper. Claiming personal power was a way for students to take action in their learning. The action seemed to help them to be willing to try different academic tasks. It appeared to assist them in connecting with their own effort. I began to use this theme each day as we began our work.

An Active Learner calms down inside

An *Active Learner calms down inside* began to be used with students on November 9, 2007. When I was considering how unfocused students were when they entered the classroom, I thought that this might help them to be able to be more focused for their lessons. Establishing being calm as a goal for students can have a positive effect on student effort during lessons.

This strand of the *Active Learner Mediated Language Scaffold* was referred to nineteen times during this action research project. The way that I would model this action would be to take a calming breath, by breathing in and then breathing out and bringing the calm breath down to my stomach area, where I had just put my personal power. Students would copy my example and then we would begin our work.

When students would practice calming down in the classroom after claiming their power to learn, the faces of the students would be quiet and focused looking and their ability to listen to directions seemed to be improved. Sometimes when the class would become unfocused, we would use this as a technique to calm the class and refocus ourselves. I would see students use this calm-breath technique in line when they were getting ready to come back to class. It appeared to be of assistance to students in terms of gaining scholarly focus for academic work. A comment made by a student such as "I try my best and calm down," indicate that calming down was helpful to student focus and attempting to try academic tasks. I also observed a calm, quiet classroom as students worked on various academic tasks. Other comments such as "I calm down inside" and "Everybody was quiet so I can focus" are indicators that calming down was useful to student effort.

You are the future

Every day of the study I would enter the classroom and reflect on what I might continue to do to support student self-efficacy. One thing that I know as an educator is that students are the future and that is an important fact. I thought that it would be an important thing for them to realize. On November 16, 2007 I added You Are the Future to what we said together before we began to use our mandated scripted lessons. This part of the *Active Learner Language Mediation* is essentially feedback and goal setting. I wanted students to know that they in fact, were the future and responsible for carrying the world forward to the next generation. I also wanted my students to set that saying in their minds as a goal everyday.

The motivational words, *"You Are the Future!"* is a form of language mediation that guides students to integrate this important concept into their thoughts. It is important for students to know that their work in the classroom serves a meaningful purpose. Several comments made to me by students over the course of this study were, "I know that I am the future and it really matters what 1do. Also, I know I am important to life." Another student comment was, " 1focus because I know I am the future and I am important to life. Also it is more quiet and it helps me learn," and another comment made was "I focus on There were now three parts to the *Active Learner Mediated Language Scaffold* being used daily in my practice. Students seemed to have improved their academic efforts. 1 noticed that overall, students appeared to be more on task during the lessons.

As the days progressed in this action research project, I kept reflecting on my observations from each lesson. 1wondered what else 1could add to what we were doing on a daily basis that would add to building student self-efficacy. When I saw students enter my classroom 1 would observe many of them with sleepy faces. Some times they would be yawning and rubbing their eyes and often they would have an expression of unfocused thinking. As I thought about my work with students it occurred to me that visualizing opening up their beautiful minds might be a good mental action. This strand of the language mediation was goal setting. It was the teacher's goal to have students open their minds to the different learning tasks that they needed to try and do.

An Active Learner opens their mind

On December 7, 2007 I started to add the theme An Active Learner Opens Their Mind. There were sixteen references to this during the course of this action research project. A comment made by a student that made me aware that this might be supportive of student effort was "One thing that helped me learn was opening my mind." Another comment that indicated that this might be helpful to student learning was "The thing I liked best was to calm down and open my mind." There were now four working Active Learner Mediated Language Scaffold parts in use on a daily basis.

- An Active Learner claims their power to learn.
- An Active Learner calms down inside.
- An Active Learner opens their mind
- You are the future!

Everyday before we began our scripted Open Court language arts lesson, we would repeat the above phrases. Then we would begin our lesson. For me, this created an intensity, from the necessity to observe all of my language arts students with objectivity and clarity of purpose. How was I supporting their self-efficacy? Were the four statements that we were making on a daily basis prior to our district mandated language arts lesson sufficient to make a difference in student performance?

As students entered my classroom, I began to notice, they looked forward to using the Active Learner language mediation before the lesson started. They appeared ready to try the learning task. Their books were open to the correct page and they were either ready to read or write as directed by me.

An Active Learner sits up straight

There were still students that had classroom focus issues. A number of students were in the habit of propping their heads in their hands and lying on top of their desks. It seemed difficult for them to focus and try the academic tasks that we were working on, specifically the Open Court Language Arts scripted mandated lesson. I was observing these behaviors on a daily basis. As I reflected on my practice and support of student self-efficacy in the classroom, I thought that adding sitting up straight would be beneficial to students.

Sitting up straight is part of teacher feedback. On December 13, 2007, this theme was added to what we were saying on a daily basis before we started our lessons. This theme was referred to fourteen times in my observations notes. Sitting up straight was described and modeled by the teacher. Backs were to be straight and feet were to be under the student's own desk. Student's eyes and faces were to be looking toward the front ofthe room where the teaching would be coming from. Hands were not to be supporting heads and students were not to be lying on top of their desks.

Five parts to the *Active Learner Language Mediation Scaffold* were now used on a daily basis with students. So far what was developed and being used on a daily basis was:

- An Active Learner claims their power to learn.
- An Active Learner calms down inside.
- An Active Learner opens their mind.
- An Active Learner sits up straight.
- You are the future!

As I followed my research notes, I discovered that this Active Learner Language Mediation was being used on a daily basis. This language was being used before regular lessons began and it fell into the region of teacher management. More importantly, I noticed that students were not lying on their desks as often and they would remember to not prop their heads with their hands. They appeared to be more alert overall and if on occasion students forgot these behaviors, I could say to them, "Please be an Active Learner" and they would remember to sit up straight and try to focus.

Students gave me feedback on the use of this theme by telling me that using this theme helped them to sit up straight and work faster. A student told me that sitting up straight helped them to focus.

The *Active Learner Mediated Language Scaffold* continued to be used with students through April of 2008. The Active Learner Scaffold was used in this form with students through April of 2008. I was finding the Scaffold was helpful to me in working with students in the classroom. I could monitor student work in progress and if a student were unfocused, I would quietly remind them to be and Active Learner. This usually was enough to help them to refocus their academic efforts. There were students in my class that responded neutrally to the Active Learner Mediated Language Scaffold. Some of them would have difficulty focusing even with this teaching tool. I would have to consider some other alternative to assist these students in their work.

An Active Learner tries to do the learning task and An Active Learner knows it is their responsibility to learn:

My reflections continued to lead me to thinking about self-efficacy and supporting it during my teaching. I wondered what else I might do to enable students to have a connection with their own academic effort. Part of building self-efficacy is based on outcomes of performed tasks. I wondered what else could be added to the *Active Learner mediation* that would assist this. Connecting to self and personal effort is a skill that takes time to become aware of. One beginning part of learning this skill is to become aware that trying to do something helps you to learn how to do the attempted task (Gredler, & Shields, 2008).

My reflections on my teaching practice also led me to consider that young students need to be aware of their own responsibility to learn and it is also important to try and do different learning tasks. These two important concepts were added to the scaffold between April 7th and April 11th. These additional *Active Learner Mediated Language* concepts were added to the scaffold between April 7th and Apr 11th . They were as follows:

- An Active Learner tries to do the learning task
- An Active Learner knows that it is their responsibility to learn!

These *Active Learner Mediated Language* concepts were added late in the action research project. These both fell into the region of language mediation. "A major role of speech is that it contributes to the semantic and systemic construction of the child's thinking (Gredler & Shields, 2008). With only one more month of school, I continued to observe student effort and see if I could observe student's behaviors that were self-efficacious in nature. There was one indicator of self-efficacious behavior that was reflected in a substitute teacher's note left for me. Her note to me was that my plans for her were very detailed. She also said that "This is a wonderful class and I will be happy to substitute again if you ever need a substitute teacher." There was also another note left for me from another substitute teacher. It said, "The day went by so quickly. No problems. We had a great time. Loved being in your classroom." This reflects to me that the students were able to perform in a satisfactory way for these teachers, even in my absence, demonstrating that the behavior came from themselves.

I also became more explicit in my language with the students in my class; the students in my class became more explicit in their performance in class. This means that that what I observed is that they calmed down, sat up straight, tried to do the learning task and in general seemed to demonstrate a more focused effort in their academic work. My reflection also allows me to see that explicit and purposeful language can help students to connect with the self-efficacy process which is language in part and skill in part.

Go Active Learners

As I continued to reflect on what I observed students doing during my lessons, I wondered if there was anything else that might strengthen their willingness to try to do the various academic tasks that they were asked to do. One more concept that I thought would help student effort was, Go Active Learners! I thought of the many times I would see students sitting in a way that would indicate to me that they were thinking of doing something other than what we were working on in class. A student might be gazing out of the window, shuffling a small piece of paper on the top of their desk, or mindlessly tapping their pencil on their desk. It was my intention to motivate students to be active in their learning efforts and Go Active Learners! was a motivational call to personal action for students. This part of the language mediation was a goal set by the teacher. The teacher wanted students to be motivated to actively learn. It was a simple, direct way to inspire academic action.

The Active Learner Mediated Language Scaffold was now being used every day before the scripted mandated language arts lesson. The scaffold was:

- An Active Learner sits up straight.
- An Active Learner calms down inside.
- An Active Learner opens up their mind.
- An Active Learner claims their power to learn.
- An Active Learner tries to do the learning task.
- An Active Learner knows that it is their responsibility to learn.
- Go Active Learners!
- You are the future!

One comment that a student made about being an Active Learner is that they liked being able to focus and they knew they were the future and stated "I am important to life." Another comment that a student made to me was that they liked being an Active Learner because they thought that they could do almost anything. The school year was over June 6th, 2008.

My observations from my journal notes indicated to me that most students were more engaged in trying to complete academic tasks. They were either engaged in peer exchange, or trying to complete various academic tasks independently. Students with a neutral response to the Active Learner Mediated Language Scaffold would struggle with their work and 1 would try and assist them using other teaching strategies. Feedback from parents indicated to me that the mediated language was supportive of the diverse cultures that were present in my class. Parents approved of the language and thought that it gave their children positive guidance in their classroom behaviors.

Different parents would come to me and ask for a copy of the student print out of the *Active Learner Mediated Language Scaffold*.

My daily reflections on my teaching practice and student effort in this language arts block made me aware that these themes may assist students to become aware of positive classroom behavior. What I observed from my research journals is that there appeared to be a connection from the mediated language, to the meta cognitive process, to self-efficacy and back to the mediated language. Below I provide a graphic illustration of this process. What I observed over the course of the action research project was that the *Active Learner Mediated Language Scaffold* led students to attempt different academic tasks. The student attempt to try different tasks helped them to grow in various academic skills that we were practicing. There appeared to be a connection between the use of the *Active Learner Mediated Language Scaffold* to the attempt and to students thinking of the *Active Learner Mediated Language Scaffold* without being prompted by me. I observed a student grabbing a hand full of personal power and centering himself quietly and then he began to furiously write. He had made a meta cognitive, higher level thinking connection with the Active Learner Claims Their Power to Learn and motivating himself to begin his academic writing. The use of the theme provided the student with the meta cognitive association that he made for himself and his claiming of his power to learn. After claiming his power to learn, he tried to perform a writing task. I observed this student working this way later in the academic day. We were not using the Active Learner Mediated Language Scaffold in our work at that time. I saw the potential for this language to be helpful to learners in elementary classrooms.

What I observed during the course of this action research project is that the language guided students to more on-task performance. Their personal behaviors were more scholarly and their mindset appeared to be more focused in academic tasks. The following chart shows the loop from language mediation to student effort and the finally support of student self-efficacy.

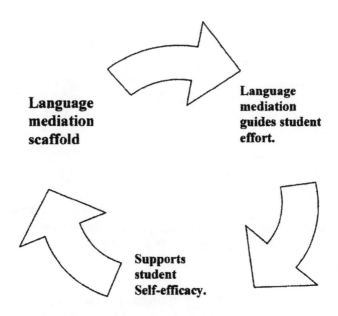

Language mediation scaffold

Language mediation guides student effort.

Supports student Self-efficacy.

There is a loop from the scaffold to the student attempt to the connection with self-efficacy. Self-efficacy is supported positively depending upon the psychological matrix of the individual student. The language of the Active Learner Mediated Language Scaffold is constructed in a way that positively influences support student self-efficacy.

Discussion

The analysis of the daily observations would indicate that the *Active Learner Mediated Language Scaffold* offers support to on-task behavior in the classroom. What the mediated language appears to support is the growth of students ability to have a set of academic behaviors that guide them to more productive academic effort and is supportive of them in their academic journey through the school system. The *Active Learner Mediated Language Scaffold* and subsequent development of the *Active Learner* mediated language that resulted from this action research project suggest that these are helpful tools in setting a scholarly mindset for students. The *Active Learner*

Mediated Language Scaffold suggests a support of self-efficacy. Analysis of my observation journals reveals that my practice appears to support student self-efficacy. The month's that fall short of positive on-task behavior were either at the beginning of the study before the Active Learner language had been used for any length of time or was before a significant school break or right after a long academic break. The following chart shows the analysis of my journal notes as follows:

On Task Behaviors

Over the course of the action research project I saw on task behavior start at about 50% and by the end of the study on task behavior occurred around 80% of the time. On task behavior was defined by students attempting to do their academic work.

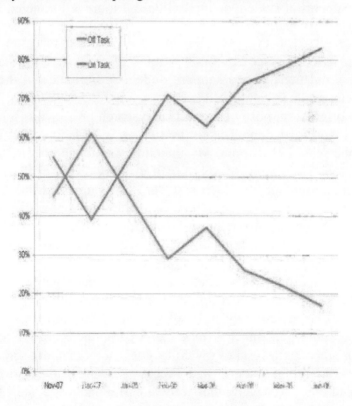

Chapter 5

Discussion & Action Plan

My overall research question was as follows: How did my teaching support student self-efficacy? Within this main question, I focused more specifically on what ways my practice supported student self-efficacy through the following mechanisms:

- Lev Vygotsky's language mediation. (Gredler & Shields, 2008).
- Feedback opportunities (Narciss, 2004).
- Teacher expectations (Rubie-Davis, 2006).
- Goal setting (Page-Voth, 1999).
- Support of student culture (Gillard, Moore & Lemieux, 2008).

Since self-efficacy is "rooted in the core belief that one has the power to effect changes by ones actions" (Pajares & Bandura, 2006, p.3), how did my practice support student self-efficacy in the public school classroom?

The original purpose of this action research project was to analyze my teaching practice in terms of the support of student self-efficacy in the public school classroom. My intention was to find a way to guide students to a stronger sense of self-efficacy. The incident which occurred so long ago in which a student communicated that knowing he was the future made him believe in himself, pointed me in the direction of student self-efficacy. This made me aware that I wanted as many students as possible to have a positive learning experience in my classroom.

The *Active Learner Mediated Language Scaffold* that resulted from this action research project appears to be a helpful tool in assisting students to set a scholarly mindset for their academic work. It is a strand of management that may be incorporated into a teacher's teaching practice. Several of my colleagues inquired about some of the student growth that students had experienced under my instruction. I mentioned that I was using the Active Learner language and I thought that it might have helped students to be more focused in their academic efforts. I suggested that they mention to parents that the student was learning in an Active Learning classroom.

I think that observing students become more aware of their own learning process should be enough of an indicator for me to realize that this action research project has given me some valuable insights to student learning. As I consider additional implications of the scaffold I realize that the different themes fall into different areas of metacognitive processing. An Active learner sits up straight is a physical action that students take. An Active Learner calms down inside is affective in nature. It is internal and quiet. An Active Learner opens their mind is a cognitive mental act. An Active Learner tries to do the learning task is also cognitive in nature. The use of language guides the students to various physical and mental acts (Gredler & Shields, 2008). The use of the language guides the students to make the metacognitive connections that support a student's "self-efficacy beliefs" (Pajares, 2006).

During the course of the study I received parent feedback that indicated to me that parent's from diverse cultural backgrounds approved of the language of the Active Learner Themes. I found the language supportive of student learning and effort. It was simple and students could understand what they were expected to do as a learner. Further action on my part will result in the use of a power point presentation that I will present to my Elkhorn School colleagues when the administration can schedule its presentation. I will also turn into my district office a copy of my thesis and a copy of the Power Point presentation. I will make myself available to share this information with any educator in my district that would be interested in seeing it. I will further extend my willingness to share this project with the CSUMB credential program, should it be of interest to them in the training of new teachers.

This action research project adds to the body of studies that examine self-efficacy. The Active Learner Scaffold and Active Learner Themes are promising tools for educators. As promising as the scaffold appears to be, there are limitations that this action research project must address. One is that the time of the project was limited to slightly over one semester of an academic school year. A long length of time in the research phase would have provided more information to the research project. Another limitation that this study must address is that I have had a lifetime interest in self-efficacy. My own interest in self-efficacy through out my lifetime may have influenced the way that I interpreted this study.

I find myself asking more questions about the use of this *Active Learner Mediated Language Scaffold*. Further research on the support of self-efficacy in the elementary school classroom would require a more expanded time frame in spite of the Active Learner Mediated Language Scaffold's educational promise. Further academic research and analysis of its use would have to be done to determine its value in a quantitative study.

Appendix

On Task and Off Task Behaviors During the course of the study

11/9/2007	5 on task behaviors	4 off task behaviors	On task = 55%	Off task = 45%
12/2/2007	5 on task behaviors	8 off task behaviors	On task =39%	Off task = 61%
1/14/2008	18 on task behaviors	15 off task behaviors	On task =55%	Off task = 45%
2/1/2008	10 on task behaviors	4 off task behaviors	On task =71%	Off task = 29%
3/3/2008	5 on task behaviors	3 off task behaviors	On task =63%	Off task = 37%
4/1/2008	14 on task behaviors	5 off task behaviors	On task = 74%	Off task = 26%
5/1/2008	7 on task behaviors	2 off task behaviors	On task = 78%	Off task = 22%
6/4/2008	10 on task behaviors	2 off task behaviors	On task = 83%	Off task = 17%

References

Bandura, A. (1997). Self-Efficacy: The Exercise of Control. New York: Freeman and Company.

Bandura, A.et al. (2006). Self-Efficacy Beliefs of Adolescents. Greenwich, Connecticut: Information Age Publishing.

Bong, M. (2005). Within-Grade Changes in Korean Girls' Motivation and Perceptions of the Learning Environment Across Domains and Achievement Levels. Journal of Educational Psychology, 97(4).

De Haan, E. (2006). Action learning in practice: How do participants learn? Consulting Psychology Journal: Practice and Research, 58(4)..

Gilliard, J. Moore, R. & Lemieux, J. (2008). In Hispanic Culture, the Children are the Jewels of the Family: An Investigation of Home and Community Culture in a Bilingual Early Care and Education Center Serving Migrant and Seasonal Farm Worker Families. Retrieved from the world wide web 7-17-20089:27 a.m. http://ecrp.uiuc.edu/v9n2/gilliard.html

Gredler, M. & Shields, C. (2008). Vygotsky's Legacy. New York: The Guilford Press.

Narciss, S. (2004, p. 11-16). The impact of informative tutoring feedback and self-efficacy on motivation and achievement in concept learning. Experimental Psychology, Vol. 51(3). Accession Number zea-51-214 Digital Object Identifier: 10.1027/1618-3169.51.3.214

Page-Voth, V. and Graham, S. (1999) Effects of goal setting and strategy use on the writing performance and self-efficacy of students with writing and learning problems. Journal of

Educational Psychology, Vol. 91(2). http://search.ebschost .com/login.aspx'?direct=true&db=pdh&AN=edu-912-230&site=ehost-live (29 June 2007).

Pajare, F. & Bandura A, et al. (2006). *Self-efficacy beliefs of adolescents* Greenwich, Connecticut: Information Age Publishing, Inc.

Pastorelli, C. & Barbaranelli, C. & Rola J. & Rozsa, S. & Bandura, A. (2001). The structure of children's perceived self-efficacy: A cross-national study. European Journal of Psychological Assessment, 17(2), pp. 87-97. Accession Number: jpa-17-2-87 Digital Object Identifier: 10.1027/10155759.17.2.87

Rubie-Davies, C. M. (2006). Teacher expectations and student self-perceptions: exploring relationships. Psychology in the Schools. 43(5). www.interscience.wiley.com.

Scholz, D., & Gutierrez D., & Sud, S. & Schwarzer, R., Is general self-efficacy a universal construct? Psychometric findings from 25 countries. European Journal of Psychological Assessment, 18(3),2002. pp. 242-251.

Stipek, D.J. (1981) Children's perceptions of their own and their classmates' ability. Journal of Educational Psychology, 73(3).

9625795R00052

Made in the USA
San Bernardino, CA
22 March 2014